THE GLOW

THE GLOW

AN INSPIRING GUIDE
to *Stylish Motherhood*

WRITTEN BY VIOLET GAYNOR, PHOTOGRAPHY BY KELLY STUART

Foreword by Cynthia Rowley

STEWART, TABORI & CHANG, NEW YORK

Published in 2014 by Stewart, Tabori & Chang
An imprint of ABRAMS

Library of Congress Control Number: 2013945649

ISBN: 978-1-61769-068-6

Editor: Rebecca Kaplan
Designer: Rachel Willey
Production Manager: Erin Vandeveer

The text of this book was composed in Brown, Miller Display, and Lucia.

Printed and bound in the United States

10 9 8 7 6 5 4 3 2 1

Stewart, Tabori & Chang books are available at special discounts when purchased in quantity for premiums and promotions as well as fundraising or educational use. Special editions can also be created to specification. For details, contact specialsales@abramsbooks. com or the address below.

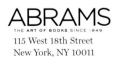

THE ART OF BOOKS SINCE 1949
115 West 18th Street
New York, NY 10011

www.abramsbooks.com

CONTENTS

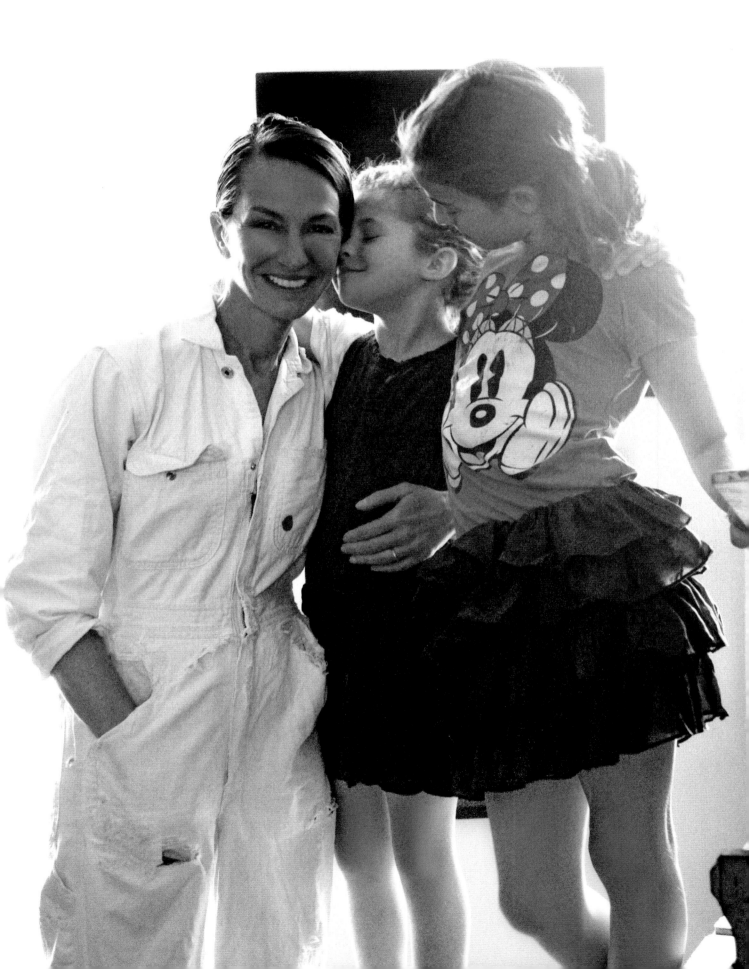

*H*aving my picture taken is my least favorite thing in the world but when my children, Kit and Gigi, and I were photographed for *The Glow*, it was easy, fun, and to this day, they are my most cherished photos ever.

Kelly and Violet have been able to capture being a mom in a way that's never been done before. The women in this book are all different, living totally different lives, but the common thread of motherhood connects them. Magical moments throughout show us it's not about the stuff; it's about the love, the relationship, and the bond.

I like to think of motherhood as a great big adventure. You set off on a journey, you don't really know how to navigate things, and you don't know exactly where you're going or how you're going to get there. There are always great surprises, and things unfold that inspire you to learn and grow.

I always found it funny that being called *Mommy* makes you feel incredibly special while on another level it's the most common name in all of human history. *Home* is another one of those terms—it's so generic, yet it has a completely different, deep association for everyone who utters it. Where you live, how you live: These are expressions of who you are at the most functional, complicated level. It's your bomb shelter, your nest, your clubhouse, and your sanctuary.

There's a connection you feel as a mom and a kind of magic in discovering who your kids are. Some aspects of their personalities are directly traceable to relatives, while other things they do come right out of left field. Like when my little one "invented" skipping backwards and I realized kids are the perfect cover for all those things you want to do but might otherwise look crazy doing as an adult . . . swinging, playing tag, hula-hooping.

It's ironic to me that as a New Yorker, where life travels at light speed, when I get home I wish I could make time stand still like the moments you'll see in this book. There's a comfort you get from reading the stories of motherhood on these pages. Every woman here feels the overwhelming joy of being a mom. The experience is universal.

—Cynthia Rowley

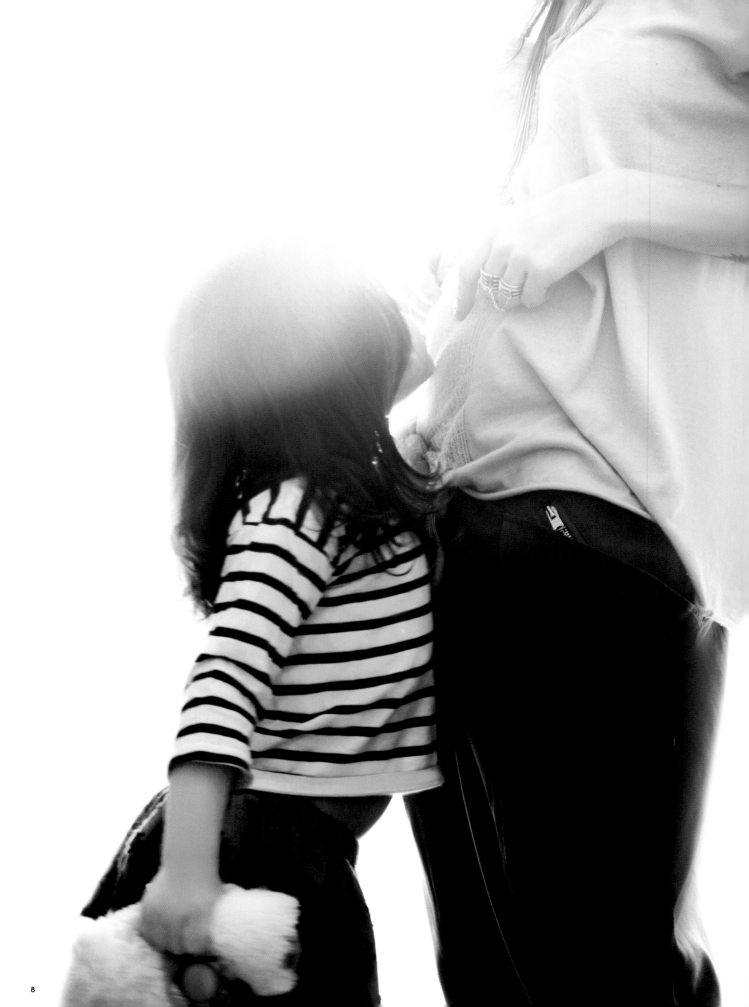

*W*hen Kelly and I first created The Glow, we were both thirty-one years old and more than a little overwhelmed by the idea of having children and how we could possibly balance motherhood and our beloved careers. For us, creating the site was a way to explore motherhood before actually becoming mothers. We put our hearts and souls into making the most inspiring guide for expectant mothers, new moms, and also women like us who were excited and a little terrified of what motherhood actually looks like—inside and out.

Kelly and I met in our late twenties while working together at ELLE.com (as photo director and senior fashion editor, respectively), and shared many striking similarities. To start, we are both incredibly passionate about our careers and have spent years working tirelessly to achieve our desired goals. Also, and not at all insignificant, Kelly and I both grew up in female-only households—we each have sisters and were raised by single moms. Women ruled our worlds. Strong, capable, empowered women at that. Despite our rock-hard role models, we both struggled with the increasingly baffling question: How could we do it all (or even attempt to)? Thriving yet demanding jobs, meaningful friendships, lasting love, thoughtfully curated homes, and effortless style?

Kelly and I realized that accomplished, multi-tasking, smart, dynamic women, who also happened to be moms, surrounded us. We started The Glow to find out how they did it. As we met, photographed, and interviewed these inspiring, super-successful women, the picture started to come into focus. The designers, stylists, actresses, and entrepreneurs we profile have opened their home and their hearts to us, and revealed their secrets to stylish motherhood.

The Glow is not about perfection, or having it all. The women in this book, and on our site, all have one thing in common—each is striving to create an inspired world for themselves and their little ones. Another thing they all possess? Power. Not only in the business sense of the word, but in their sheer strength. As every woman knows, when you become a mom, you also become a super hero overnight. The Glow represents modern motherhood—it's the delicate mix of trying to balance a passion for career with an equal passion for creating a rich home life, while still honoring the all-important relationship we have with ourselves.

When I started to write this book, I was newly pregnant. When I hit send on the manuscript, I had just started to go into labor, and now as I write this introduction, I am a new mom. Throughout the process, Kelly and I have experienced some of life's most meaningful and transformative moments. Hours before hopping on a plane to London to shoot for our book, Kelly got engaged. As we completed the book, she married the love of her life. One year later, we are wholly different women than when we started.

As with everything we do, Kelly and I have worked obsessively to bring you the very best advice and visual inspiration—whether you're a seasoned mama or just trying to figure out how to make the dream of being a working mother a reality—and we hope this guide will bring you inspiration and clarity. Two things every woman deserves.

CHAPTER ONE

Labor of Love

REBECCA MINKOFF, *designer* · TRACY ANDERSON, *fitness & health expert*

JODI FAETH, *business partner, Antique Archaeology* · CASS AND ALI BIRD, *photographer and director of The Wall Group*

YAYA ALAFIA, *actress* · HILARIA BALDWIN, *health & fitness expert* · JESSIE BAYLIN, *singer*

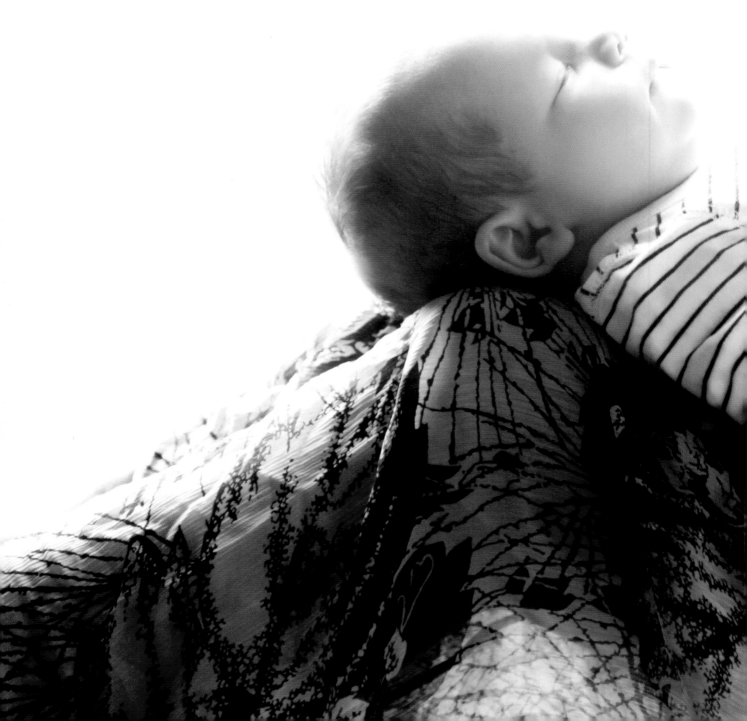

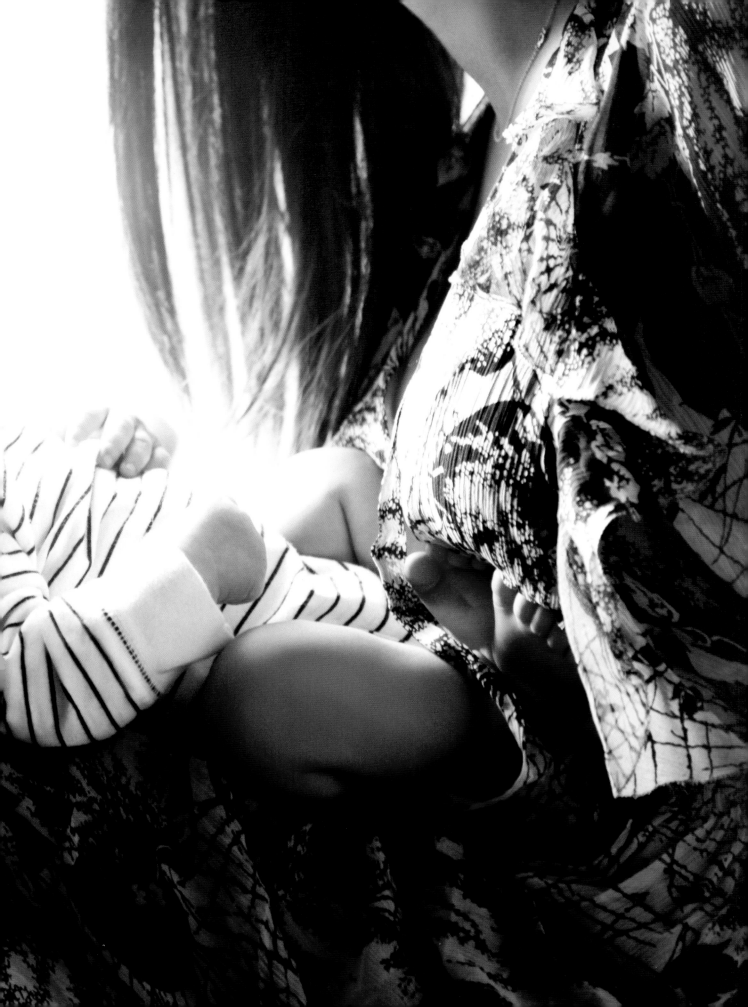

*T*here are 101 ways to give birth, or so it seems when you start doing the research. Ultimately, the path to figuring out a birth plan comes down to gut instinct (or in some cases, necessity). I come from a long line of women who labored with midwives and delivered naturally, oftentimes at home. So when it came time to decide how I wanted to bring my baby into the world, I went with what was familiar and came up with a natural birth plan, though I knew that a home birth was not for me—my cozy yet snug Manhattan apartment just didn't seem to fit the bill. In this chapter, we explore the myriad options leading up to the actual birth (doctors, doulas, and midwives, oh my!), hard-earned insights (laboring in water is not always as tranquil as you'd think), and inspiring birth stories. Each experience was powerful and perfect in its own way. Whether aided by doulas or epidurals, these entrepreneurs-turned-moms describe their path to bringing babies into the world.

But one of the greatest lessons of motherhood, surrendering control, starts before the baby even arrives. For Tracy Anderson, a shining example of perfect health, the realization that she would have to bring her daughter into the world by way of a C-section was heartbreaking at first. But after delivering a healthy baby girl, Anderson's focus quickly shifted to her number-one priority: breast-feeding, which she was able to do right away. Designer Rebecca Minkoff was determined to deliver her son sans drugs, in a hospital birthing center (to re-create the environment of a home birth, while still being surrounded by medical equipment should something go wrong). In the end, she was able to accomplish the former, not the latter. Despite more than a few setbacks, Minkoff delivered her son naturally, conquering her biggest fear.

Just like it's impossible to plan a pregnancy, planning a perfect birth can also be quite elusive. However it ends up happening, the words to describe the journey are the same: connected, euphoric, amazing, exhilarating.

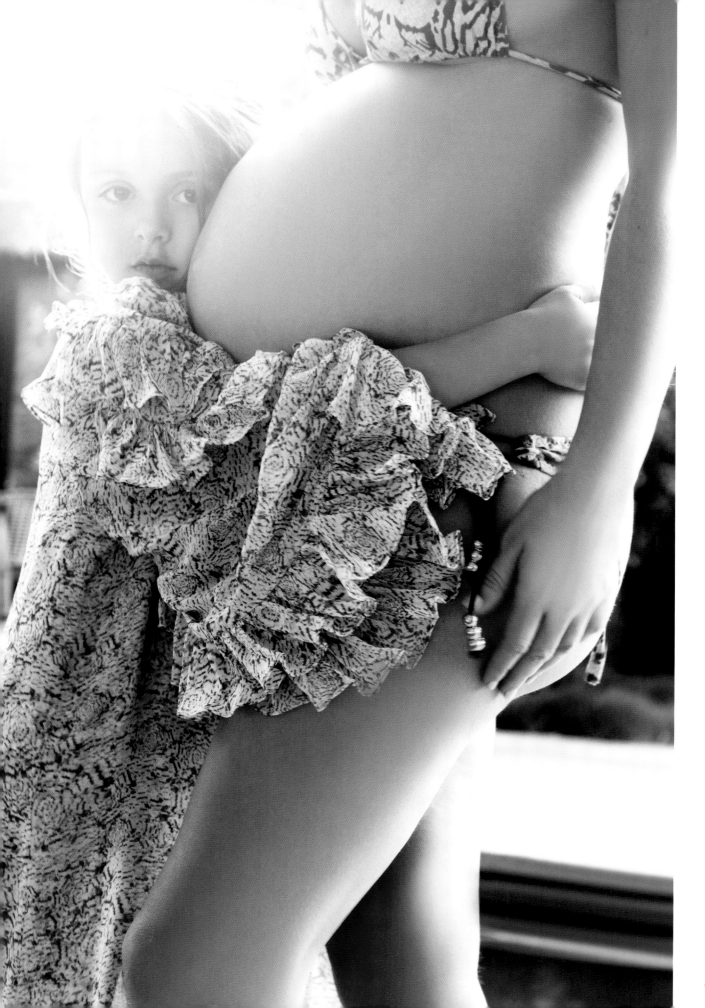

Rebecca MINKOFF

Son Luca,
photographed at three months old
New York, New York

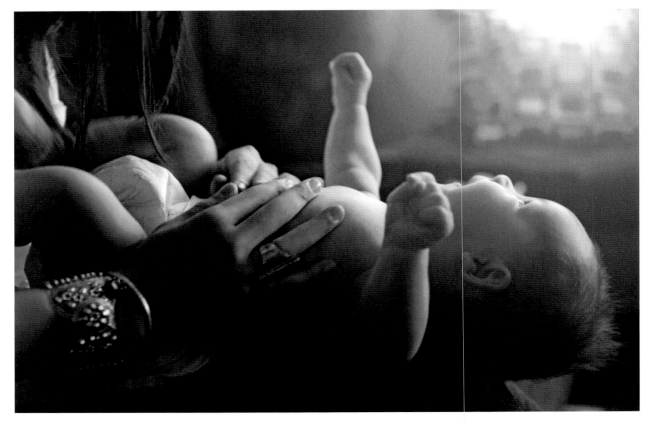

Rebecca Minkoff won the hearts of women everywhere when she introduced her now-famous, party girl–inspired "Morning After" bag. Fast-forward eight years, and the young designer is still charming the world with her must-have handbags, only now there's even more to obsess over, including her coveted ready-to-wear and footwear collections. With a gift for tapping into the desires of her loyal following, she's achieved that elusive combo of critical and mainstream success. Minkoff has approached new motherhood with the same passion and honesty she applies to her growing empire. Loving husband and easygoing son complete the perfect picture. Enviable life aside, it's the wicked sense of humor and "girl's girl" charm that make Minkoff our perennial crush.

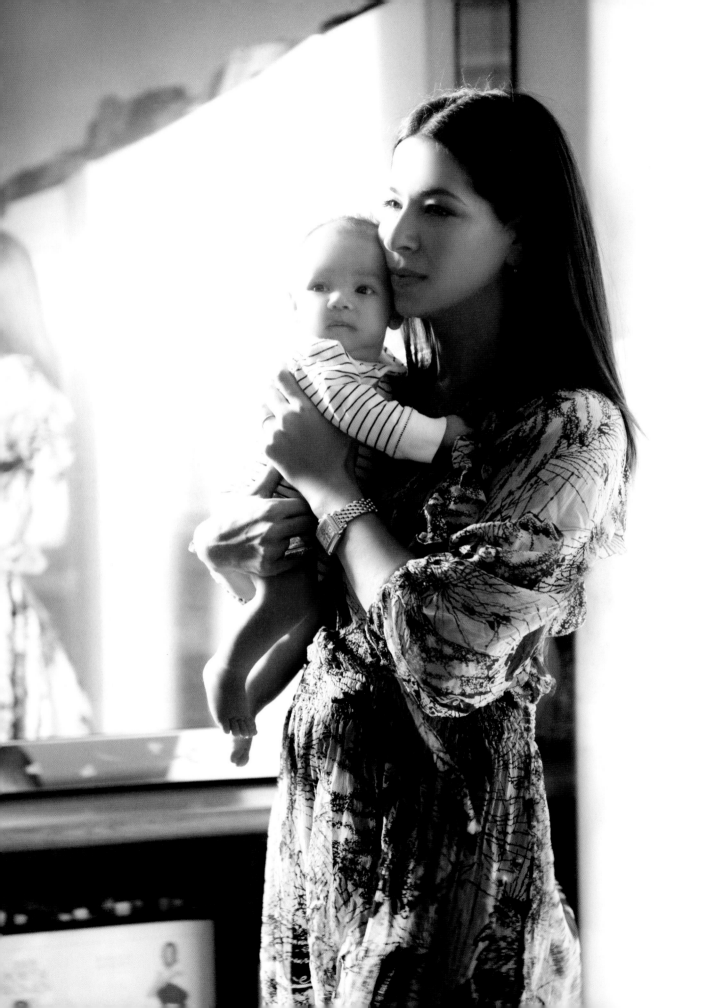

*R*EBECCA ON MOTHERHOOD: I felt really natural—it was instant. The thing that I thought would also be natural was getting Luca on my boob, but it wasn't. I was determined not to give him a bottle, but we ended up having to supplement with a little formula when he was first born.

BEST ADVICE: My mom told me to let him learn to play on his own—it makes the baby more independent and less reliant on you for all their entertainment.

HARDEST PART: Working and being a mom are now a constant pull on my heart! I'm still trying to figure out the work/mommy balance. I try to cut off the day once I get home—work stops, and I focus on my son.

PROUDEST MOMENT: Seeing Luca smile for the first time.

THE SUPPORT TEAM: I met a lot of midwives and tried to find someone who was supportive of my beliefs and that I could relate to. But I also needed to know that this person would ask for help if an emergency arose.

THE BIRTH PLAN: It was very important to me to do my best to have a natural birth. I didn't want to introduce anything that would interfere with what our bodies have been doing for thousands of years.

THE BIRTH STORY: Two days before Luca was born, I went to the hospital and was told that my fluid was low and was instructed to go home, rest, and drink water. I was also warned that I might need to be induced if my fluid remained low. I promptly went home and proceeded to drink water like a camel. I also made raspberry tea and took evening primrose to soften my cervix. When I went back to the hospital for an ultrasound, thank god I had gotten my fluid levels up and they did not have to induce me. I went home and had the strongest urge to sleep and sleep—I just couldn't get enough. I started to have Braxton-Hicks contractions, which got stronger and more intense but were not particularly painful. By midnight, they were ten minutes apart. I decided to get in the tub and relax for an hour. By the time I got out, I looked at my husband and said, "I think we are in labor."

We called our doula around one a.m., and by then my contractions were fluctuating between five and eight minutes apart. At this point, the only thing that helped was when my doula would grab the pressure points in my hands and Gavin would dig into my back during a contraction. We tried many positions; we used a birth ball; we walked up and down the stairs of my apartment (which made things come on fast and furious). This continued until around five thirty a.m., when my contractions were three minutes apart—then Gavin and my doula decided to get me to the hospital.

After arriving at the hospital, I was put on continuous monitoring right away because I had a two-vessel cord and they worry that contractions can be hard on it during labor. The only position I could handle at that point was squatting on top of Gavin as he sat on a stool. His legs were shaking, and I was howling at the top of my lungs. Then my water broke, and since there was meconium in it, my midwife wanted to hurry and get the baby out. From there, I felt a sudden need to push and got onto all fours on the bed and started pushing. Because they could not get a read on the baby's heart rate in that position, my midwife had me do a side-lying squat, which was HORRIBLE. She then began to instruct me to stop screaming and start pushing! She told me my pushes were too weak and decided to call the doctor to chat about a C-section. Upon hearing that, I finally got the hang of it and began pushing like a crazy woman! Out he came, with no tearing, and he had the best set of lungs in the room! Everyone sighed, as it had looked so grim when they could not get his heart rate on the monitor.

Luca Shai was born weighing six pounds, fourteen ounces—one week early but perfect, happy, calm, and so yummy. We achieved our goal of one hundred percent natural birth despite not being allowed into the birth center.

What my husband found most amusing was that in our birthing class, when we were taught about screaming and moaning, I said that is the one thing I would not do during labor—at the time, I just didn't see the need. Needless to say, moaning bloody murder was very helpful in getting me through!

THE BIGGEST SURPRISE: That I did it—I conquered the scariest thing in my life. Also, I wasn't prepared for how strong my mother-bear instinct would be. I wanted Luca at my side and didn't want him going anywhere at all unless my husband was with him.

Tracy ANDERSON

FITNESS & HEALTH EXPERT

Daughter Penelope, photographed at eleven months old
(not pictured: son Sam, fourteen years old)
New York, New York

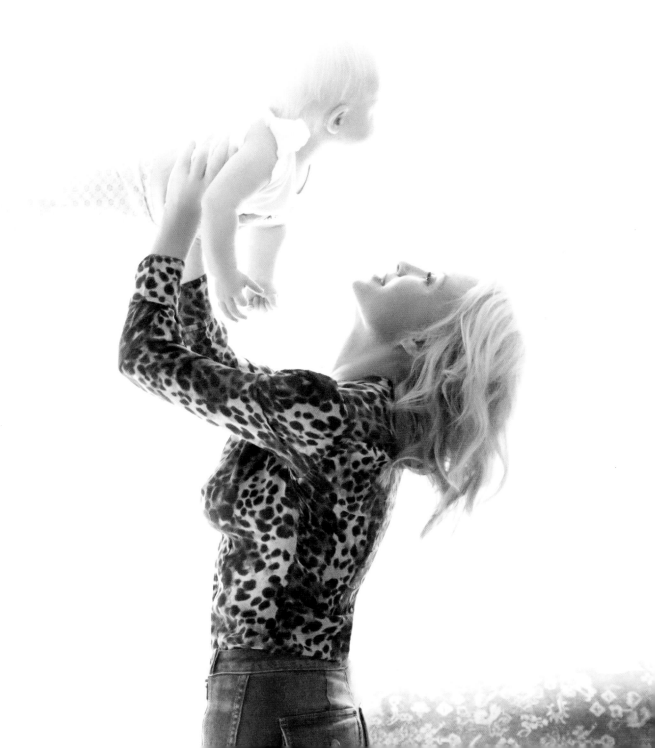

*T*racy Anderson, aka Gwyneth Paltrow's pint-sized miracle, has made it her mission to empower women through her unique brand of health and fitness. Beloved by women around the world for her shape-shifting techniques, this mother of two truly practices what she preaches. Case in point: her wildly popular *The Pregnancy Project* DVD set, which follows her during each of the nine months leading up to her daughter's birth (it's worth mentioning that many of the mamas featured in this book, myself included, swear by her method before, during, and after baby). While she's the picture of perfect wellness, Anderson is not immune to health obstacles and encountered her fair share of unexpected issues throughout her pregnancy, including undergoing a C-section. Despite some bumps in the road, Anderson believes everything worked out the way it was supposed to in the end, and she credits her fourteen-year-old son with helping her through. From that experience, she realized that her little boy was turning into an impressive young man. Job well done.

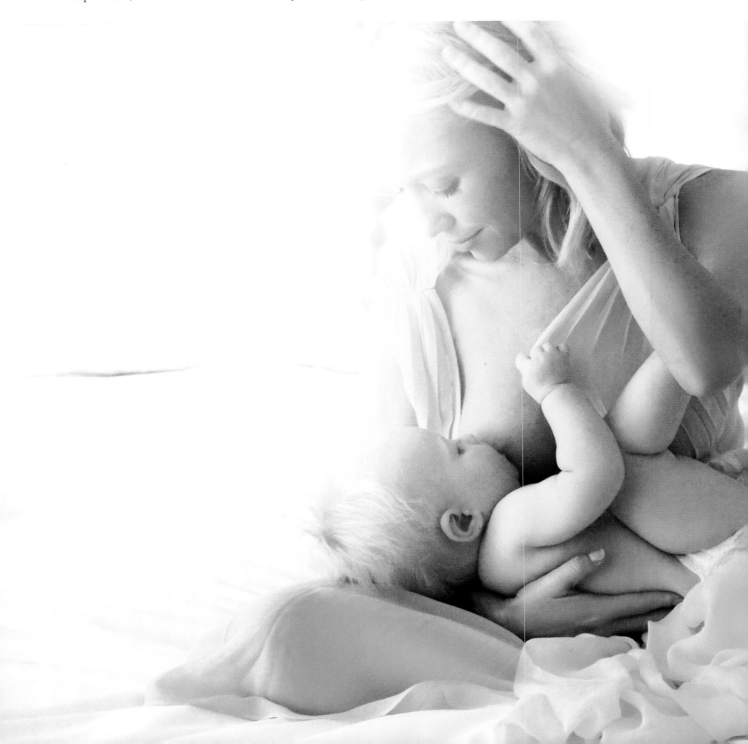

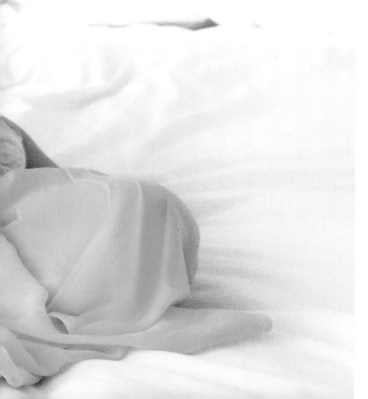

TRACY ON MOTHERHOOD: I loved everything about being pregnant—I was born to be a mom.

BEST PART: It's the most whole, complete feeling of love, and it's the easiest thing to sacrifice for. You know, anything can happen in the world, but if I can just be with my kids, I'm absolutely in pure joy.

HARDEST PART: The worry and need to protect them. I love and respect them as individuals from the moment they come into the world, but I want to make sure that I give

them the safety that can help them develop into people who can take care of themselves. The nanny thing is also really tough. I did not have a nanny with Sam, but I have had one with Penny, which has been really difficult. As mothers, we need to really, really listen to our gut, and never, ever be convinced otherwise.

MAMA INTUITION: I have a fourteen-year-old and a one-year-old. Because there's such a large gap between my two kids, I was shocked the second time around to realize how much we have in us as women and how strong our instincts are. I was thirty-eight years old this time, and I'd lived a long life in between my two pregnancies, yet I experienced the same kind of powerful instinct and feeling and intuition. From the second you become pregnant, you're responsible for this other person, and I'm so connected to that responsibility.

THE SUPPORT TEAM: Trust is a big issue for me, so I had to find the doctor I trusted most, first and foremost. I am a very natural mother, and a natural parent, but this is one of the times when I do trust the medical community. There are so many options and so many ways to bring a baby into the world, but for me the main thing is feeling one hundred percent comfortable—that's the only thing that makes me feel natural about it. The doctor I ended up choosing to bring Penny into the world is an amazing woman—she was cool, calm, collected, and understood every single one of my needs.

THE BIRTH PLAN: I delivered naturally with my son, but I had to have a C-section with my daughter. When you go through the process of getting ready to have the baby, your body is gearing up, and you're so focused on bringing the baby into the world, and you almost feel like delivering naturally is the last effort of earning your part in bringing this beautiful life into the world. So when I heard that I was going to have to have a C-section, I was really taken aback. It just seemed like a "procedure," which felt so weird to me. Since it's major surgery, my main concerns were about breast-feeding. So I asked a lot of questions, because I had to make sure I got to the point where I felt comfortable. And sometimes I asked the same questions over and over so the doctors understood the seriousness of it.

THE BIRTH STORY: The C-section was such a weird experience—they set up that big screen, and you're numb from the waist down, and even though you're awake, you feel far away from what's happening. I will never forget my son's

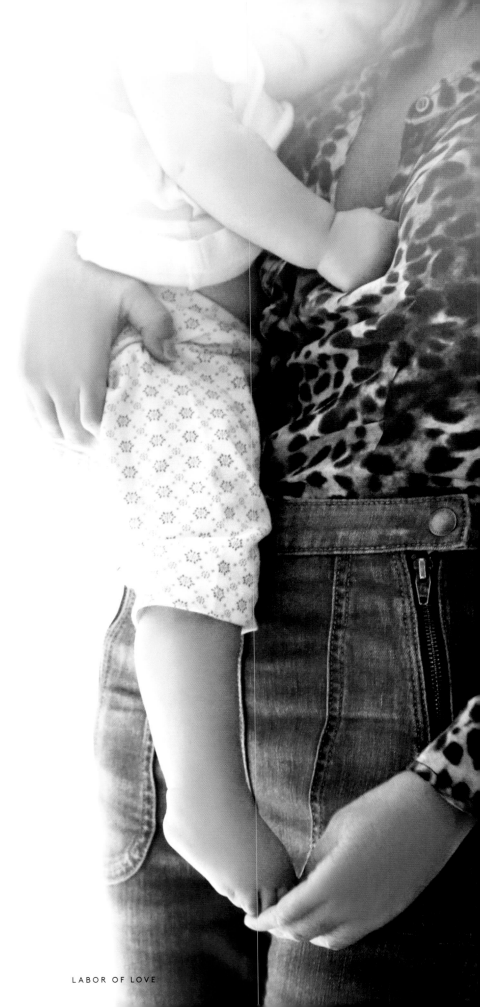

face as he left the operating room right before I went into surgery to have Penny. He said, "OK, Mommy, I love you," and as the door was closing, he looked at me every second until it was completely closed.

SHINING STAR: My son actually helped me through my pregnancy the most. Because I was diagnosed as high risk while I was in California, I was told I wasn't able to fly anymore and couldn't return to New York. So Sam left his school (and all of his friends) to come be with me and get tutored for the rest of the year. He truly helped me so much with the gestational diabetes. He was amazing. It made me so happy to realize what an amazing man he'll be when he grows up.

AFTER THE BIRTH: My main concern, because of the C-section, was about being able to breast-feed right away. Luckily, I was able to do it immediately with no problem. But I was very determined and told every nurse, every attendant, every single person around me that breast-feeding was the top priority for me, so please make sure that the baby and I stay together and that I get to nurse her right away. They really listened, and Penny never had to leave my side. I follow attachment parenting completely. I plan to nurse Penny as long as she wants. I let my son wean himself, and he nursed for three years (but by the third year was nursing only at night). It's the best thing for me and my kids.

ON THE DAY PENELOPE WAS BORN, I WAS . . . Completed, connected, devoted.

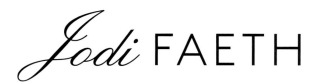

Jodi FAETH

Daughter Charlie, photographed at one year old
(not pictured: son Kyle, twenty-four years old)

Leiper's Fork, Tennessee

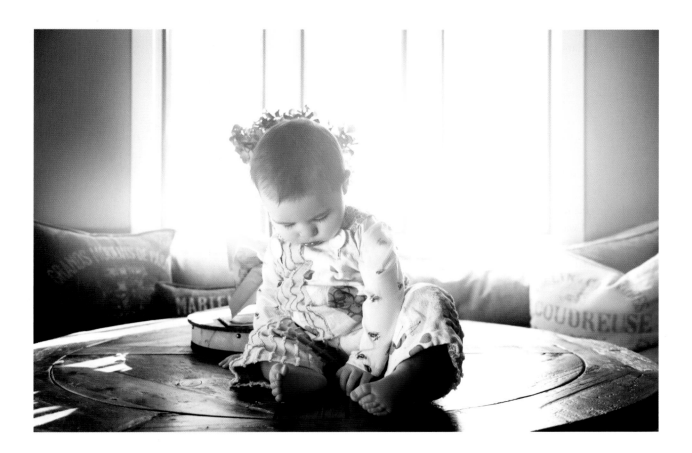

As mom of a twenty-four-year-old and a one-year-old, Jodi Faeth has the kind of highly honed mama instincts that come only from a lifetime of mothering. Walking into the sprawling Tennessee home she shares with her husband (and *American Pickers* star Mike Wolfe) is like traveling back in time—there are vintage motorcycles in the living room and a classic 1960s VW van parked outside. But it's the home's enveloping warmth that's most striking. After a difficult labor and angst-filled year of multiple surgeries to correct a cleft palate, the proud parents are thankful for every healthy day they get to spend with baby Charlie.

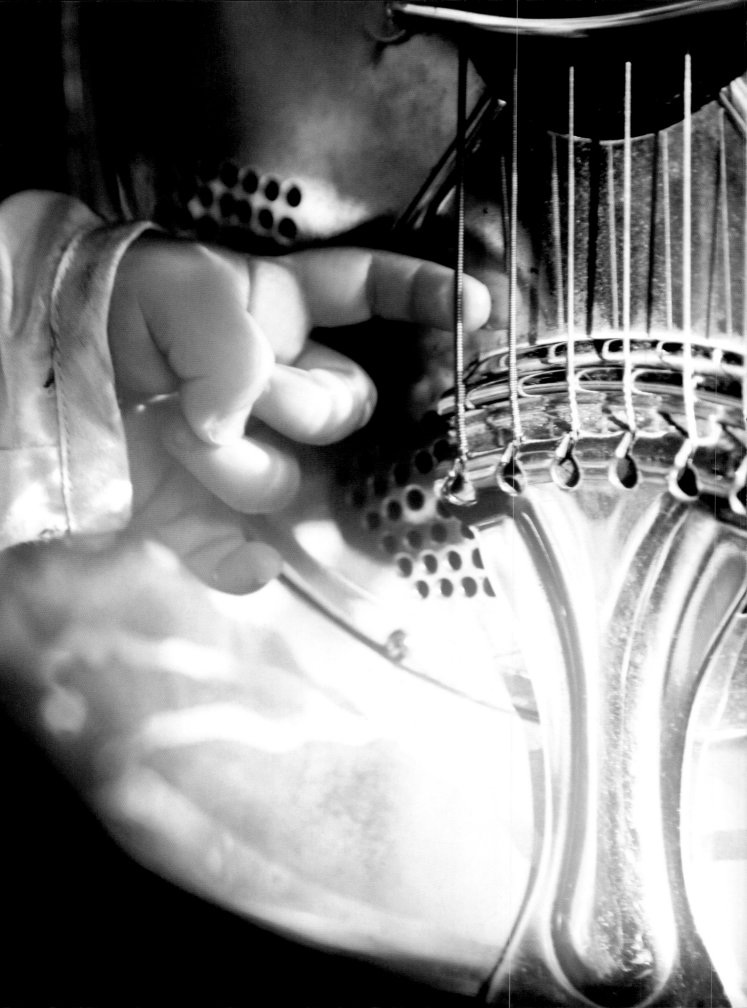

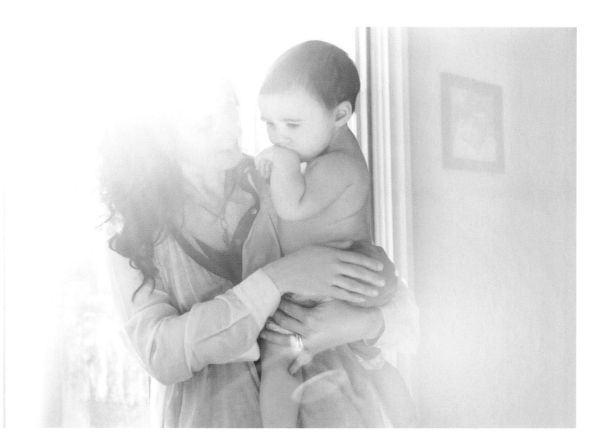

*J*ODI ON MOTHERHOOD: I was more scared to become a mother again at the age of forty-one than when I had my son, Kyle, twenty-four years ago. The first time I was so young, and I also didn't know any better. Back then, I didn't research strollers, cribs, and schools. I keep reminding myself that my son turned out just fine—and the most important thing I did with him, and I will continue to do with Charlie, is spend time with them without an iPhone, iPad, or other distractions.

MOST HUMBLING MOMENT: While I was in recovery from my C-section, my husband showed me a picture of my son holding Charlie for the first time, and Kyle had tears in his eyes. We had gotten the girl we had dreamed about, and my son got the sister he never knew he wanted but fell so in love with. He later told me that he never expected to feel the way he does about his sister and that he will be there for her always.

BEST PART: The wet kisses, and the blueberry pancakes in my hair. Kids make you remember your own childhood and how fun being silly can be. Not everything has to be so serious.

LIFE LESSONS: I am instilling strong will and confidence in my daughter every chance I get! Being born with a cleft lip and palate, Charlie will have to overcome some obstacles with speech and having a scar above her lip. I tell her every day what a strong, beautiful girl she is on the inside and out. I want my children to be givers, not takers, as that is the greatest expression of self-worth. That is how I will know I did my job right.

THE BIRTH PLAN: I didn't have any drugs the first time around, so I wanted everything as natural as possible with Charlie. We had no idea she would be over nine pounds and that I would be in labor for twenty-eight hours before a C-section was necessary.

THE BIRTH STORY: After finding out about Charlie's condition in utero, we were devastated initially but quickly decided we could handle her birth defect and would embrace it and be strong for her. We were already so in love with this girl that nothing could have changed how we were feeling. When we returned to the doctor, we were advised to take all sorts of tests because once they find one birth defect, your chances of other syndromes are high (and I was forty-one years old at the time). I said no to any and all tests—I knew in my heart Charlie would be healthy, and I decided that I would not let any stress enter my otherwise healthy pregnancy. She was born January 30, 2012, weighing nine pounds four ounces. After my surgery, when I finally got to hold her and count all ten fingers and toes, all the worry was finally over. She was perfect, and we were ready to take on any obstacles she would face. We bonded immediately. She made a fist and shook it at my husband. I think she was mad about how long the whole thing took. At that moment, all of my dreams came true.

AFTER THE BIRTH: Feeding is usually the biggest issue for babies born with clefts. She lost weight right off the bat, but we figured out a solution by cutting a Y in the bottle's nipple. Mike and I were so proud of her, we told everyone about her cleft and even shot her baby announcement photo with it. We had two surgeries the first year she was born.

Those were tough. We are a team, and we stayed together every night at the hospital. Charlie is a strong girl—she even surprised the surgeons and got to go home early. We realize how fortunate we are that we had the resources to get Charlie the best doctors. We became ambassadors of Operation Smile, an organization that provides lifesaving surgeries for children in countries where the resources are not available. Charlie inspires us to be better people, and through this I hope the three of us can make a difference.

ON THE DAY CHARLIE WAS BORN, I WAS . . .
Relieved, exhausted, complete.

ON THE DAY CHARLIE WAS BORN,
MIKE WAS . . . Strong, amazed, complete.

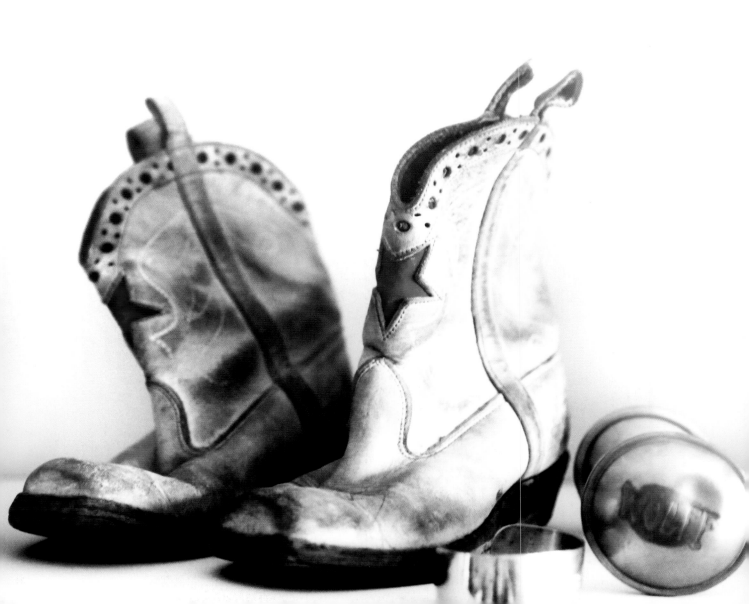

Cass and Ali BIRD

PHOTOGRAPHER & DIRECTOR OF
THE WALL GROUP, RESPECTIVELY

Son Leo and daughter Mae, photographed at
six and three years old, respectively

Brooklyn, New York

With their infectious energy and overwhelming love for each other, Cass and Ali Bird's Brooklyn home is so fun and inviting, you don't ever want to leave. There are art projects in the works at the dining room table and nightly dance parties in the living room (a mix of new and old-school hip-hop is always in heavy rotation). As one of the most sought-after fashion photographers, Cass travels the world shooting for J.Crew, the *New York Times Style* magazine, and *Vogue*, while Ali is a director of the highly respected fashion and beauty agency The Wall Group, which represents talents such as Rachel Zoe, Kate Young, and Jeanne Yang. Both have embraced motherhood with such passion and vigor, it's easy to see why their children seem like the happiest kids on the block.

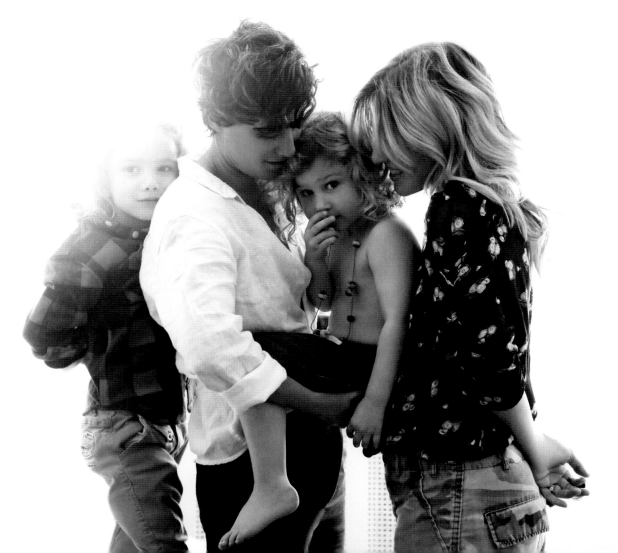

Cass

CASS ON MOTHERHOOD: It is all very humbling to me—I am not a natural.

HARDEST PART: Brushing their teeth after reading ten books and telling five bedtime stories.

BEST PART: Being witness to their beauty.

FAVORITE PART OF THE DAY: In the morning, they both wake up so differently: Mae like a live wire bursting with energy and creativity, Leo like a soft kitten, cozy and tender.

THE BIRTH PLAN: While I was pregnant, I got really into the Ina May books on midwifery. I really wanted to connect with the woman primate inside. I loved being pregnant—I connected to my feminine side for the first time and really felt a strength that was new to me.

THE BIRTH STORY: My labor was fast and really intense—it was only six hours with Pitocin and no epidural. Leo was tiny (four pounds, ten ounces), so he came out quick!

THE SUPPORT TEAM: I worked with a great OB, who was referred to us by a friend. In hindsight, I would work with a midwife for a less medical approach to childbirth. I also had a doula—I wouldn't think of childbirth without one.

AFTER THE BIRTH: The experience was so magical and powerful—I was really high on life for a few days. Then I crashed pretty hard for a few weeks with postpartum blues—the adjustment was quite drastic. Learning how to build a community to support and grow this new person has been the biggest learning experience yet.

ON THE DAY LEO WAS BORN, I FELT . . . Connected, excited, focused (all qualities that I would rarely call myself).

ON THE DAY LEO WAS BORN, ALI WAS . . . Connected, supportive, loving (and nervous).

Ali

ALI ON MOTHERHOOD: I grew up thinking my parents' word was law and the final say. Soon after becoming a mom, and now as the kids are getting older and challenging us daily, I understand that my parents were making up the rules as they went along and just trying to do their best, just as we are.

HARDEST PART: Finding balance.

BEST PART: The feeling of having grown extra hearts inside my body to accommodate the overwhelming and total love I have for these angels. It is the biggest blessing I can imagine to have these souls come through us, and to have the chance to grow and learn from them every day is profound.

FAVORITE PART OF THE DAY: I cherish telling Mae stories before bed, after we've read books. Every night she says, "Tell me a story" and falls asleep as I make up fantastical tales about a family of ice cream cones or a fairy ninja and her trusty dog, Fluffy. With Leo, I love the hour before his bedtime, after Mae is asleep, when we play cards, Monopoly, or whatever he is currently obsessed with. It's a time where I connect with him and we talk about the day. And I live for our family dance parties and "family hugs," where we each pick up a kid and have a group hug.

THE BIRTH PLAN: After seeing Cass deliver with an OB, I decided I wanted to work with a midwife. I loved having all of my checkups at home and having my son, Leo, sit with us and listen to his sister's heartbeat. I wanted to be balls-to-wall and try a home birth, but my neurotic Jewish side was too scared in case something should go wrong. So I compromised and chose to use a midwife and deliver at the hospital.

THE BIRTH STORY: I labored at home for twenty-four hours before going to the hospital! I had lots of back rubs and encouragement. Since it was right after Christmas, my doula was in Washington, DC, and had to make the winter drive back to get to us. She arrived around seven p.m., and we left for the hospital at eleven p.m. Once there, I did have some pretty scary complications, and I looked at Cass's face, from what felt like underwater, and I saw her go white with fear, and I could tell that all was not well. The realization that many women die during childbirth was not lost on me then. I was so grateful for the care I received and that they were able to stabilize me and help me through the process.

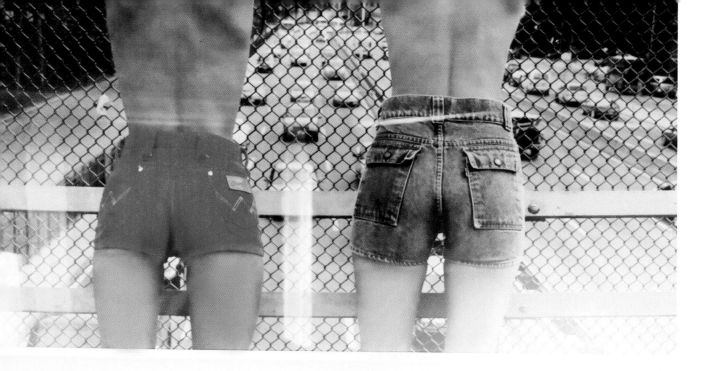

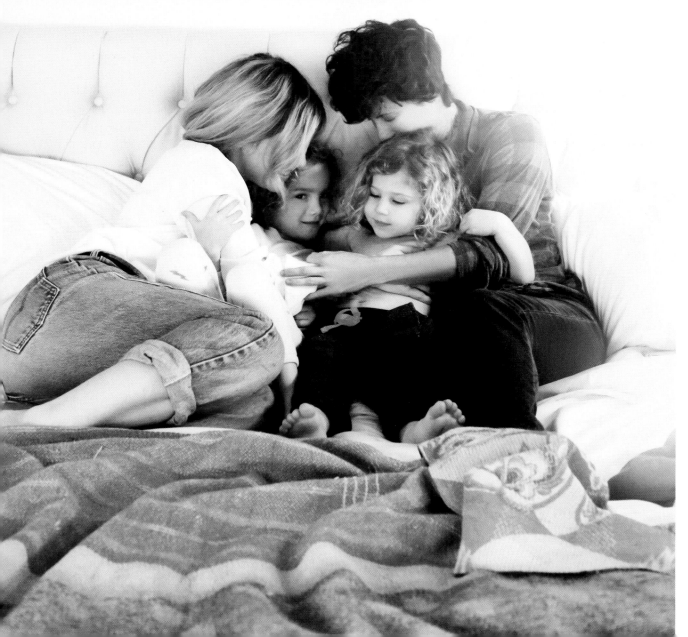

Cass was my rock. When I was in the throes of labor while still at home, she and my doula took me for a night walk around our block. I was in so much pain, and she stopped me, pointed up at the moon, and said, "Honey, right now there are thousands of other women giving birth under this same moon—you are not alone." That one sentence helped me through the rest of my labor and delivery, which ended up lasting around thirty-six hours.

AFTER THE BIRTH: I loved being pregnant. Everything about it agreed with me. Even though we think we're done with having kids, we still fight over who would get to be pregnant again—we both loved it.

ON THE DAY MAE WAS BORN, I FELT . . .
Joy, fulfilled, like a warrior.

ON THE DAY MAE WAS BORN, CASS WAS . . .
Present, solid, my angel.

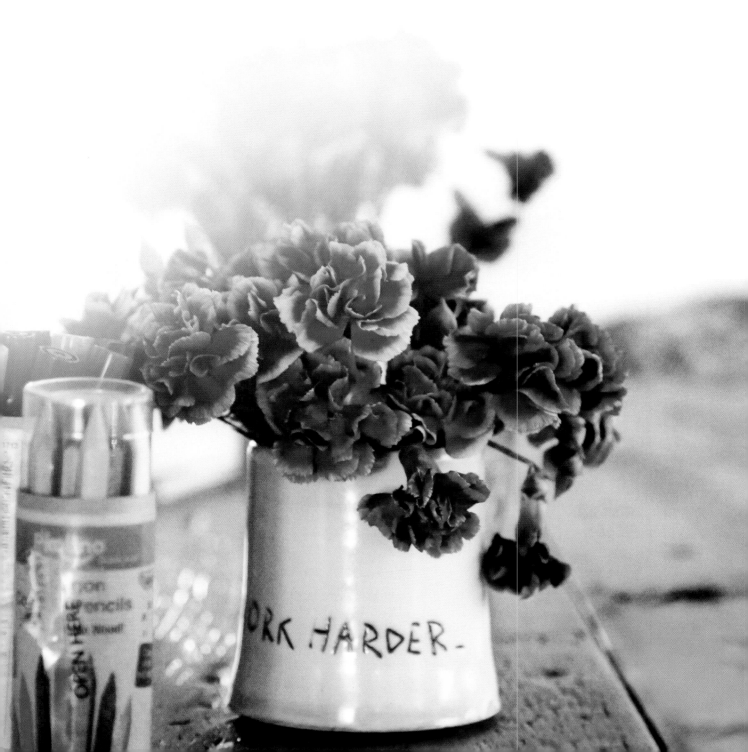

Yaya ALAFIA

Photographed at six months pregnant

Brooklyn, New York

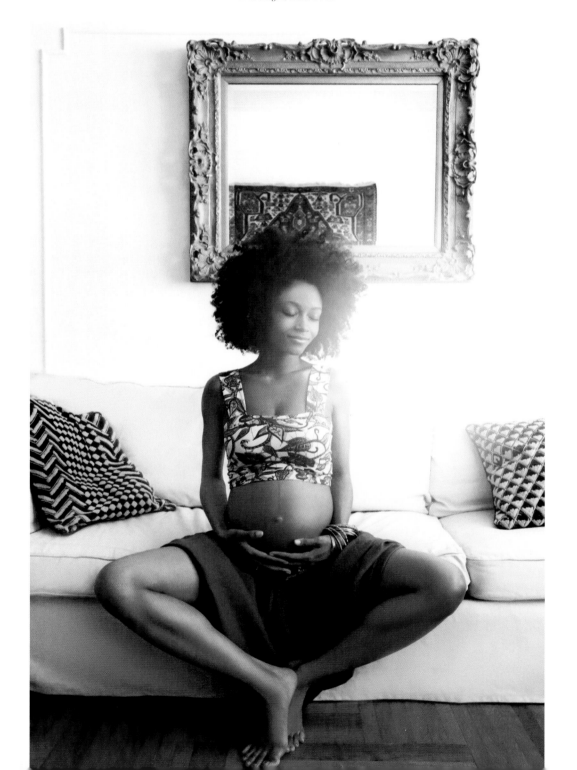

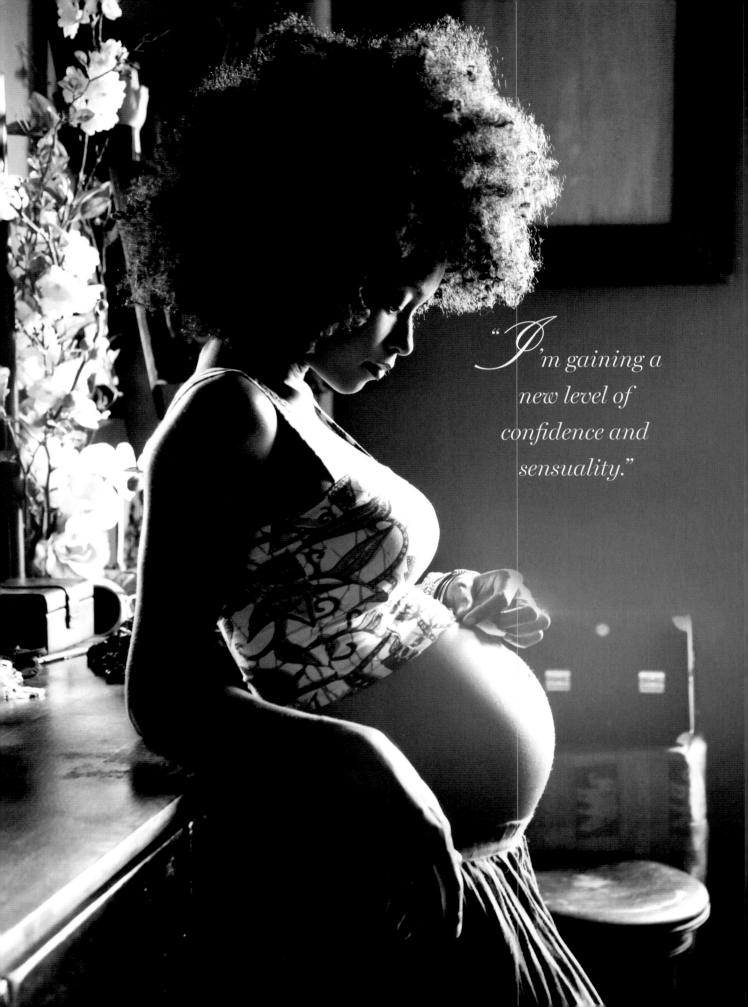

"I'm gaining a new level of confidence and sensuality."

*Y*aya Alafia has the kind of magnetic personality that makes you instantly feel like you've known her forever. It's her infectious spirit, openness, and shining-from-within beauty that have made her an in-demand young actress. When she's not on movie sets with Oprah, this born-and-bred New Yorker can be found advocating for women's maternal health-care rights and working on her very own documentary about birth in America. At the time of our shoot, Alafia was six months pregnant and eagerly awaiting the arrival of her first child. With her at-home birth plan firmly in place, this soon-to-be mom has embraced pregnancy with every fiber of her being. "I feel like I'm stepping into a new dimension of womanhood and settling into my power."

MOST TREASURED ADVICE: Let go of fear and surrender to the sensations of labor. Ride with the waves, rather than against them, and be expressive. Talking about issues in relationships, with either partners or family members, can help clear up emotional blockages and facilitate labor. I'm working on these things now!

FAVORITE PART ABOUT PREGNANCY: I'm gaining a new level of confidence and sensuality.

HARDEST PART ABOUT PREGNANCY: I was nauseous and vomiting all throughout the first trimester and a bit into the second. It's also an adjustment being so vulnerable to the comments, assumptions, and traumatic birth stories of all kinds of people, whether I know them or just meet them on the subway.

THE GROWING BUMP: As a naturally slender girl, I'd always looked forward to growing up, getting pregnant, and gaining the weight that I'd heard so many women complain about not being able to get rid of. Here I am, grown, pregnant, and carrying small—actually like my mother did with her firstborn: "all belly." I have let go of expectations and am just nurturing and enjoying watching my body go through this amazing journey!

MOST SURPRISING: I had no idea that in planning my own child's birth, I would become so passionate about women's and babies' rights during childbirth, and become involved in the fight to change legislation around hospital and insurance policies.

ON PREGNANCY AND MARRIAGE: I like to refer to "us" being pregnant and to the baby as "our baby," instead of "mine." Obviously, women do the hardest work, but I feel that men should also feel included, important, and empowered by the birth. I am grateful that I am able to be open about my feelings, to talk about every single thing with my husband—even if it would normally be TMI. Pregnancy is a time when he needs to know the details of what I'm going through—from bodily functions to emotions and everything in between. I already feel our marriage strengthening and our connection deepening, preparing him to be the most supportive birth partner and father possible.

MOTHERHOOD INSPIRATION: I find that I'm inspired by mothers I see on the street, on line at the DMV, wherever mothers and babies or toddlers are where the balance between structure and freedom is tested. I notice confident, happy babies and watch the parents to see what they're doing. Of course, my own mother is my first amazing role model, but I am also blessed to have been given a wonderful mother-in-law whose style obviously worked well enough for me to want to marry the product of her hard work. Her patience, playfulness, and generosity are wonderful examples for me.

THE BIRTH PLAN: Birthing at home is the right choice for me and will help me get in the proper mind-set to surrender and allow my baby to birth itself through me, the way we've been doing it since the beginning of time. While I am very grateful for modern medicine and its benefits when necessary, I am still young and healthy, and so far, my wonderful midwife sees no reason that I should not be able to have a normal birth. I feel most comfortable with the decision to do it at home, probably in water.

Hilaria BALDWIN

Photographed at eight months pregnant
New York, New York

Long before Hilaria Baldwin became pregnant with her first child, the renowned yoga guru followed a healthy life-style that included an all-vegan diet and daily workouts. Pregnancy only enhanced her desire to live in a constant state of mindfulness. Baldwin kept an enviably cool demeanor by working out every day (walking, swimming, and Physique 57 are all part of her regular routine), even through her ninth month of pregnancy, and taking time for herself. She credits the experience with giving her "a deeper strength" than she ever thought possible.

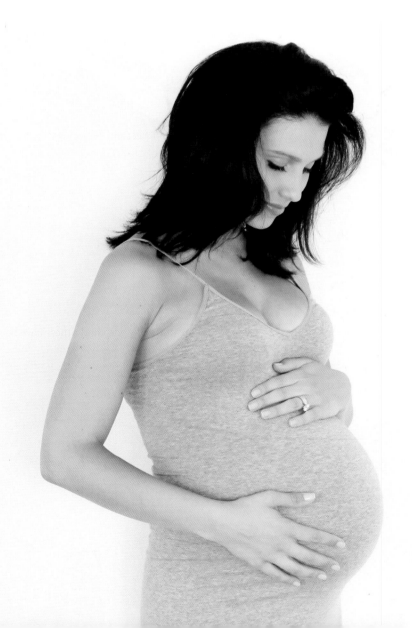

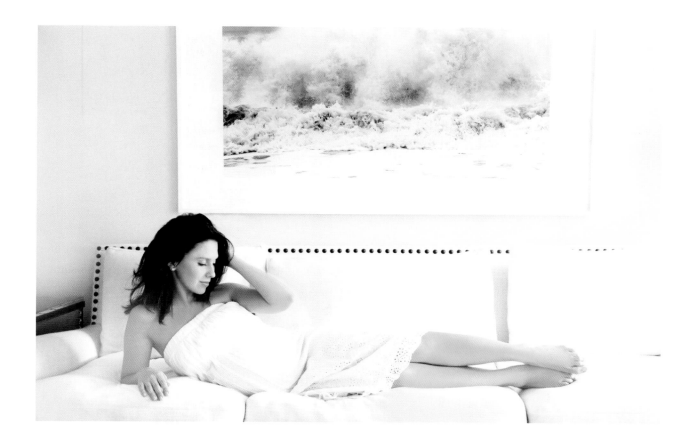

MOST TREASURED ADVICE: We all know that pregnancy can be stressful—not just the aches and the pains and the stretching, but also there is so much uncertainty and concern regarding our little one's health and growth. Humans are very good at making more humans, and we should not feel alone in the journey of pregnancy. I have been told to enjoy the process and try not to stress so much—stress will only negatively affect both of us. This has really helped me relax and realize that pregnancy is a happy time!

FAVORITE PART ABOUT PREGNANCY: Seeing her little face during sonograms.

HARDEST PART ABOUT PREGNANCY: The limits of my bladder!

ON PREGNANCY AND MARRIAGE: I think it is important to realize that while I am physically carrying the baby, both my husband and I are in this together. We are having a baby, not just me. Our marriage has only been strengthened due to the intensity of this experience. We speak a lot more about philosophy now that I am pregnant. We talk about hopes and wishes we have for our baby. We explore our most cherished values, and when we don't

see eye to eye on a certain subject, we explore it, trying to understand each other. This allows for both tremendous personal growth as we reexamine ourselves and the ability to find an even deeper love between us.

LESSONS LEARNED: About myself: I have learned I have a deeper strength than I ever thought possible. About Alec: I have learned just how caring he can be.

Maternity Must-Haves

★ Working out: daily yoga and fitness have been lifesavers.
★ My Snoogle! I can't sleep without it.
★ Eating well
★ Resting when necessary
★ Cocoa butter: I have experimented and used many different types of body butters and oils while pregnant. I have found that cocoa butter has really helped me. No stretch marks! I feel that taking time to moisturize my body is not only good for my skin but also connects me to my changing body and my baby.

Jessie BAYLIN

SINGER

Daughter Violet Marlowe,
photographed at five weeks old

Nashville, Tennessee

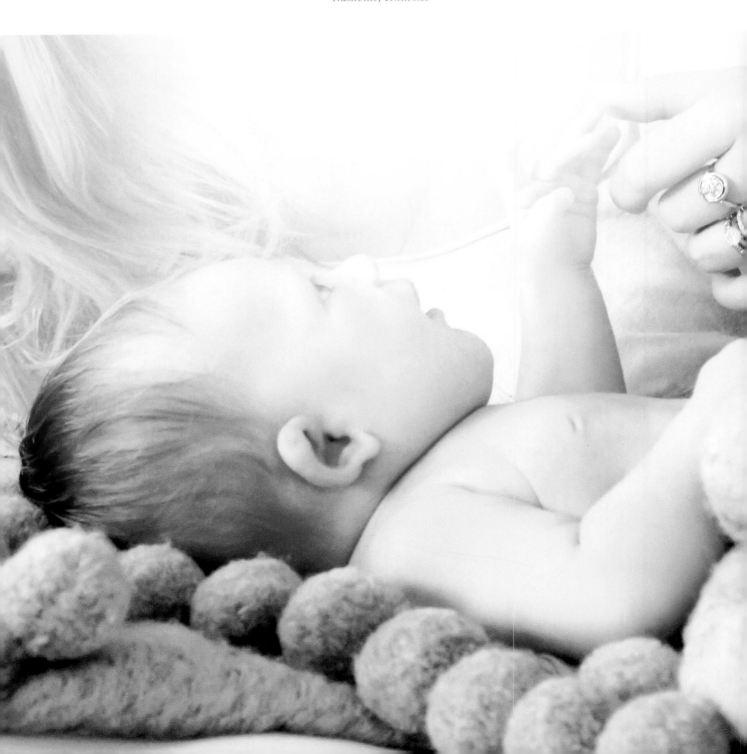

Though she hails from New Jersey, country singer Jessie Baylin oozes pure Southern charm. From the second you step into her cozy condo (a temporary abode while her 5,000-square-foot dream home was being built), you're enveloped in a feeling of calm, thanks in part to the flickering candlelight and Billie Holiday wafting from the speakers. Baylin's affable spirit and "girl's girl" sensibility only add to the home's laid-back vibe. She and husband Nathan Followill, drummer for Kings of Leon, have an equally laid-back approach to parenting. We caught up with them just five weeks after their daughter, Violet Marlowe, came into the world, and Baylin was already spilling over with words of mommy wisdom—from lessons learned from the unexpected turn her birth plan took to the delicate process of easing into her new life as a rock-star mom.

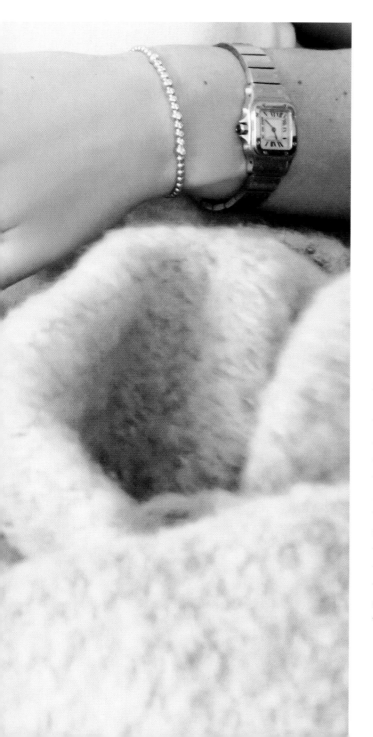

JESSIE ON MOTHERHOOD: I thought I knew love before, but my heart, soul, spirit entered a whole new dimension of love after having my daughter. The first night I spent with Violet, I thought to myself, "What am I supposed to do with this new feeling I have? How am I supposed to exist like this?"

HARDEST PART: Breast-feeding. After two horrible cases of abscessed mastitis, I had to quit—it just wasn't working for us.

BEST PART: Learning about what she needs and seeing her discover happiness.

FAVORITE PART OF THE DAY: Nothing is sweeter than our mornings in bed with Violet.

THE BIRTH PLAN: After talking to a handful of trusted girlfriends, I decided on the type of birth plan I wanted. Then I found the Midwifery Program here in Nashville, which felt like the right fit, since I wanted to have a natural birth.

THE BIRTH STORY: I had these very specific expectations of how I wanted the birth to go, and I was feeling super-disappointed when I was two weeks past my due date. I was pretty devastated when I was told I had to be induced. I instantly felt defeated, because it seemed like I was going to be missing something, and I wasn't even sure what it was exactly that I'd be missing. They had to do this treatment to soften the cervix and said it would take anywhere from twelve to twenty-four hours to start working. At around three a.m., only three hours into it, my water burst! It was exactly what I needed, to feel that flow. Then I knew I was "in it," and it all became so real and perfect.

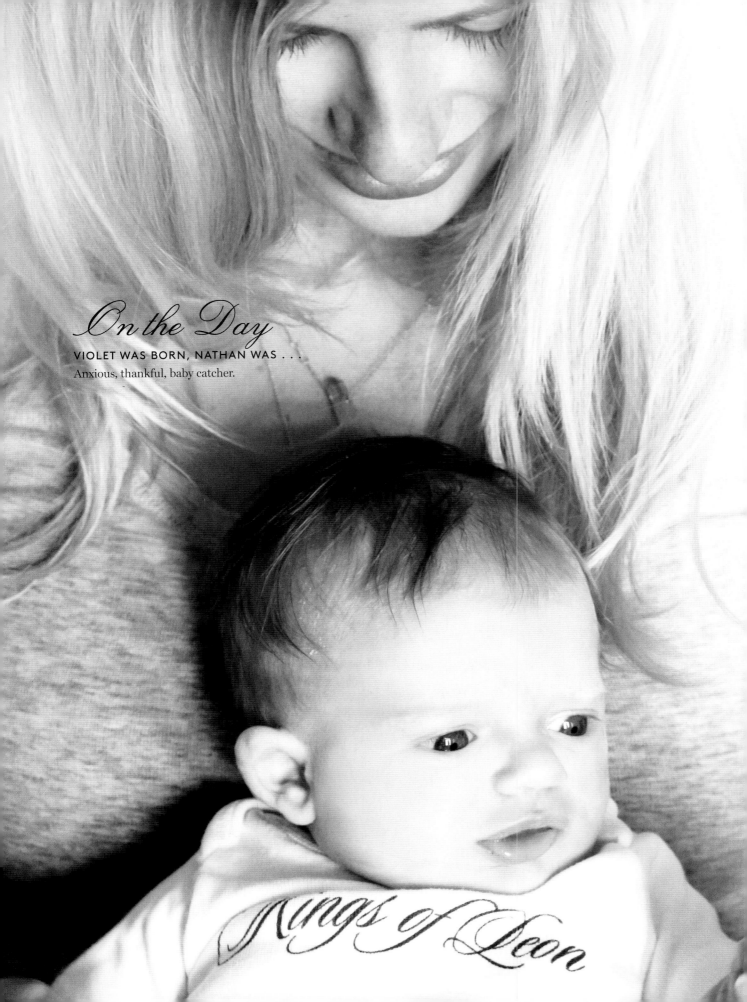

On the Day

VIOLET WAS BORN, NATHAN WAS . . .

Anxious, thankful, baby catcher.

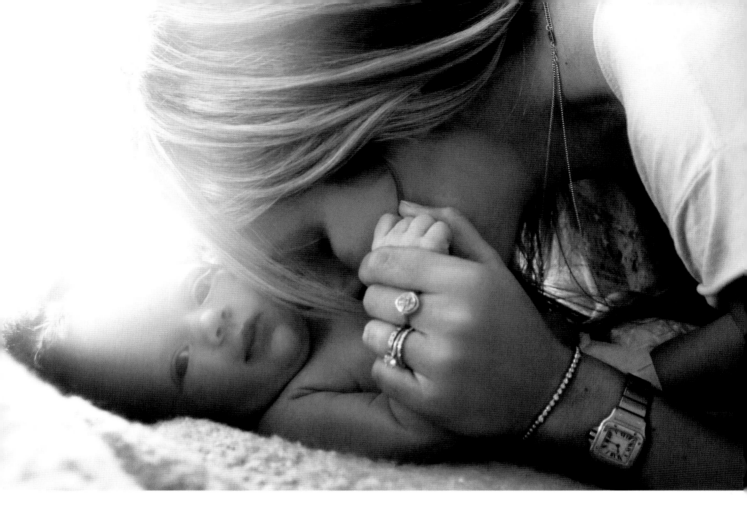

THE SUPPORT TEAM: After deciding on my midwife, I then started looking for a doula. I ended up meeting mine at a mutual friend's engagement party. She came over a couple of weeks later to give me a prenatal massage, and I asked her to be my doula forty minutes into the massage—I instantly felt like she could read my mind and was so in tune with my body.

AFTER THE BIRTH: I wouldn't change a thing! It's all the way it was supposed to be. After she was born, my husband and I had to both have patience while my hormones balanced out, and we rediscovered our relationship after this incredible event. Having a baby, this product of our love, has changed the way we look at one another. We have a lot of gratitude.

THE BIGGEST SURPRISE: It was incredible to witness the moment when I was one person, and then suddenly there were two of us. I will never forget that. Before the birth, I feared the unknown. Once Violet arrived, I knew everything was perfect and as it should be. After giving birth, I trusted the universe a little bit more.

ON THE DAY VIOLET WAS BORN, I FELT . . .
Feminine, natural, trusting.

New Mom Must-Haves

* ★ Kissy Kissy basic onesies
* ★ The Mamaroo
* ★ Travel Sleep Sheep
* ★ Anything from Tane Organics
* ★ Little Giraffe lovie
* ★ Rikshaw Design bibs and burp cloths

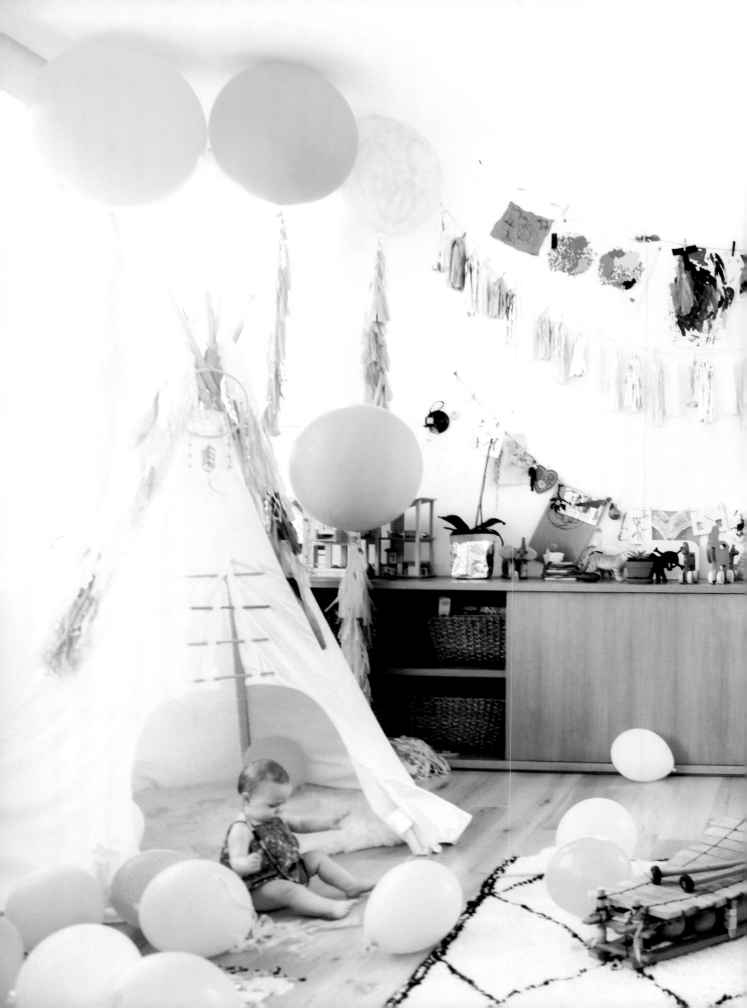

CHAPTER TWO

Treasured Spaces

JENNI KAYNE, *fashion designer* · ATHENA CALDERONE, *interior designer*

LAURA PORETZKY-GARCIA, *creative director* · JEANANN WILLIAMS, *stylist* · JADE BERREAU, *artist*

ore than any other room in the home, the nursery holds the most prom-
ise. Whether spacious or tiny, luxe or minimalist, its four walls will provide
security, inspiration, entertainment, and tranquility for your little one (not to
mention the countless hours you'll spend playing, reading, and likely sleeping there). From
almost the first moment I found out I was pregnant, I began envisioning the space I'd soon
create for my new baby. After sharing the news with Kelly, my partner on The Glow and best
friend, we immediately started brainstorming ideas. Side note: Kelly has the most amazing
collection of antiques culled from her world travels, including pieces that will be perfect for her
future little one's room. Smartly, she's always on the lookout for beautiful, one-of-a-kind items,
like the reclaimed-wood horse-fence planks with weathered blue paint she and her husband
found in Vermont. "Perfect for open shelving," according to Kelly. For the small office that
would soon become my baby's nursery, Kelly and I ruled out pink and blue, since I decided not
to find out if I was having a boy or girl. From there, the possibilities seemed endless.

Should I choose a theme, like designer Jenni Kayne did when she centered her son's Native
American–meets–safari-themed bedroom around a neon-accented teepee? For interior designer Athena Calderone, the design process started with her son's name, Jivan ("to give life"
in Sanskrit), which she turned into graphic wall art. Her decidedly unconventional approach
included covering another entire wall with an acid yellow-on-gray design she sketched herself.
From there, she cleverly mixed in her nine-year-old's favorite things—like handmade artwork
and a treasured surfboard given to him by legendary surf pro Jeremy Flores. Laura Poretzky-
Garcia took a similarly artistic approach for the design of her brand-new baby girl's Upper
East Side nursery. Not one to shy away from a challenge, the former fashion design darling and
current creative director chose wall-to-wall white carpet (the brave mom swears it hides every-
thing). Next, she accented the walls with bold art, like a floor-to-ceiling hot-pink silkscreen of
Elizabeth Taylor by Russell Young.

From clever storage ideas to a DIY-wall of family photos, these five moms each capture that
delicate balance between stylized design and smart functionality. Here you'll find their design
philosophy, inspiration, splurges (and steals!), and the biggest hoops they had to jump through
to achieve their desired look. The result: unique, stimulating, and inspired interiors for their
little ones to treasure for years to come.

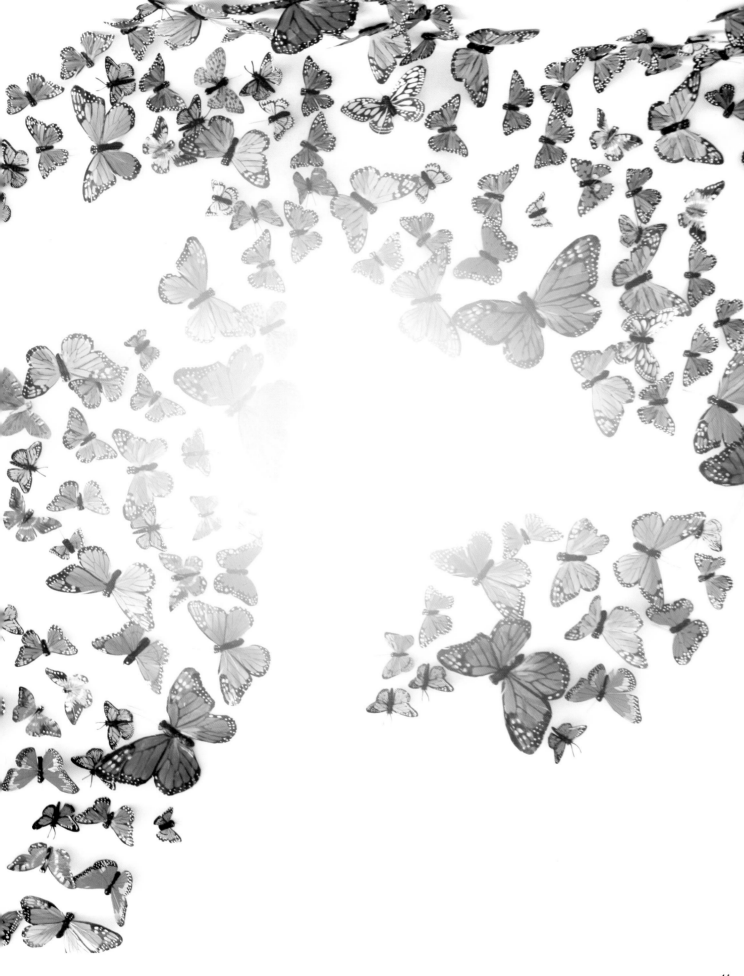

Jenni KAYNE

FASHION DESIGNER

Son Tanner and daughter Ripley,
photographed at four years and eighteen months old, respectively
Los Angeles, California

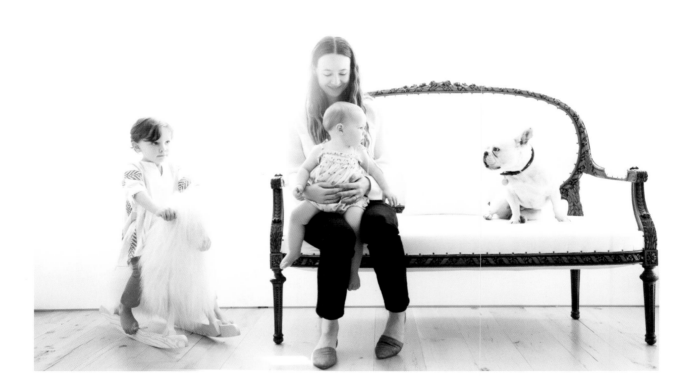

Fashion designer by day, Martha Stewart-in-the-making by night, Jenni Kayne has the kind of honed design eye usually reserved for seasoned interior designers. Not only did she design every inch of her kids' whimsical bedrooms and playroom herself, she also manages to throw a mean birthday party that adults enjoy just as much as the kids. While the California native makes it all look completely effortless (think perfectly tousled beach waves and bare feet), the young mom admits that the challenges of being a working mother are very real. "Finding balance is always a struggle for me," she admits. What gets her through? "Dinners with my girlfriends, weekends with my husband, support from my sister and parents, and a glass of wine."

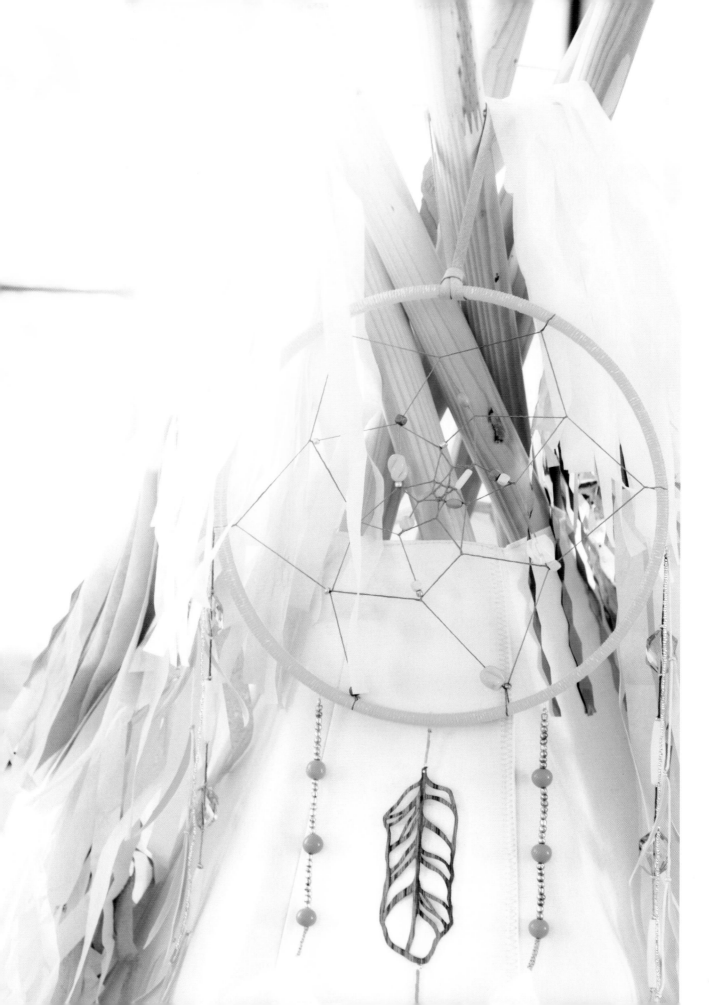

JENNI ON MOTHERHOOD: My whole world became about them the minute they were born.

HARDEST PART: Balance and patience.

BEST PART: I am in love with my kids in a way that I didn't know was possible.

FAVORITE PART OF THE DAY: Bath time. I am a bath person, and the three of us get in the tub together almost every night, while my husband sits with us. It's a special time that I won't have forever, so I cherish it.

ROOM STYLE: *Whimsical with a Grown-Up Twist*
With inspirations as varied as Native American-meets-safari, the bar at the Chateau Marmont, and French dollhouses, these playful yet sophisticated spaces—splashed with decidedly adult antiques—deliver on their bold themes without feeling kitschy.

Inspiration

PLAYROOM

I wanted it to feel like the rest of the house: clean and modern but warm and earthy, while still being fun and functional for the kids, and not too precious. I decided on pops of color but with a white base that we wouldn't get sick of. Then I found a Moroccan rug that is durable and cozy and makes people want to sit on the floor and play. I think it's all about the mix—it was important that the space feel open and organized so the kids don't get overwhelmed.

TANNER'S ROOM

When I found out I was having a boy, I wanted to create a room that was inspired by a mix of Native American and safari. The focal point is a great

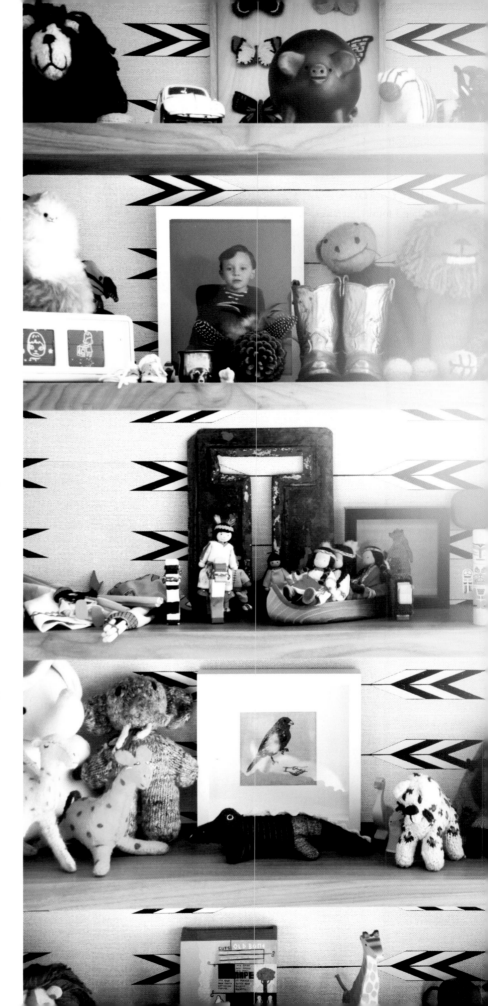

teepee with a beautiful dream catcher hanging on it, as well as other Native American–inspired art and accessories. I hung faux stuffed trophies above his bed, which plays into my safari inspiration. My goal was for his room to be bright and clean and feel like an extension of our home, but at the same time I wanted to have fun with it.

RIPLEY'S ROOM

When I found out I was having a girl, I went a little pink-crazy, which is out of character for me. I wanted my daughter's room to feel like it was straight out of Paris. I have always loved the butterflies on the ceiling at Bar Marmont and said if I ever had a girl, that's what I would do in her room. So when the time came, Maurice from Bloom and Plume sprinkled her ceiling with butterflies, and my French friend Ambre found the most beautiful wire chandelier from Paris with little birds hanging from it. Then I added a mix of modern and French whitewashed antiques, with pops of color. I put a French settee that I have had in my house for years in her room and ordered her crib from Bonton in Paris.

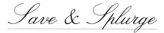

Save & Splurge

PLAYROOM
Save: IKEA kids' table and chairs
Splurge: Moroccan rug from Lawrence of La Brea

RIPLEY'S ROOM
Save: I framed beautiful bird and butterfly posters from Smallable.
Splurge: The parchment dresser from JF Chen

TANNER'S ROOM
Save: I got great linen sheets from The Company Store.
Splurge: Personalized Shirley McLauchlan blanket and Oeuf bunk bed

HOMEMADE TOUCHES: We added a chalkboard wall for the kids to draw on, and strung their artwork on jute on the wall, which looks fun and makes the kids proud.

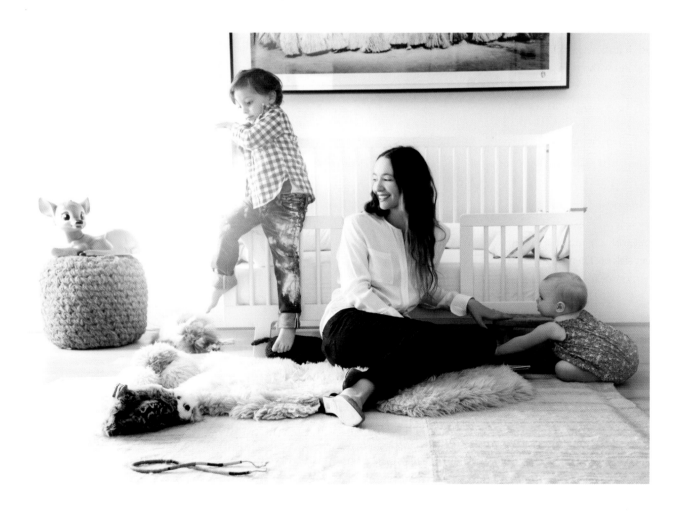

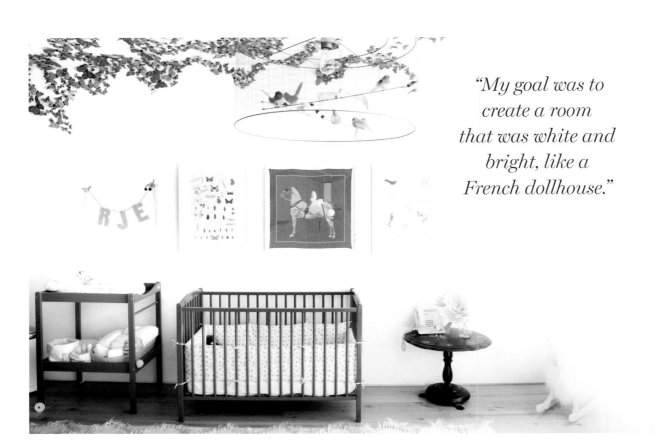

"My goal was to create a room that was white and bright, like a French dollhouse."

ABOVE: Ripley's room is filled with a mixture of new pieces, including the Bonton crib and changing table, plus some antique favorites and unexpected touches. The bright pink horse print is actually a Hermès scarf that Jenni framed. BELOW: In the playroom, Tanner proudly hangs his own artwork using clothespins. To add a touch of sparkle, Jenni mixed in a metallic garland by Confetti System.

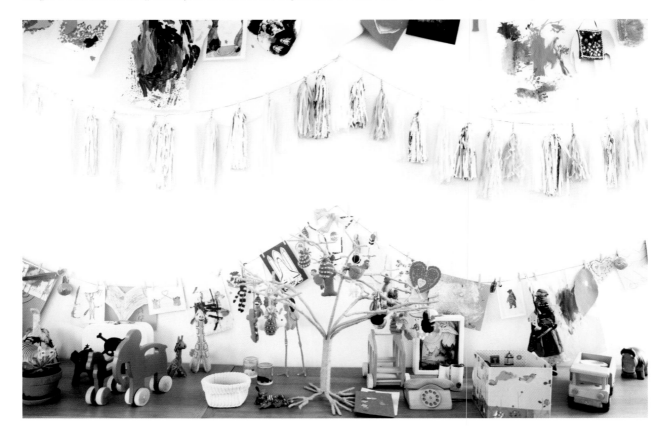

PERSONAL TOUCHES

Ripley's Room: My grandmother's self-portrait and silver jewelry box

Tanner's Room: His quilted Linda Moore portrait that I commissioned as a Father's Day gift for my husband, and his personalized Shirley McLauchlan blanket that Ripley gave him when she was born.

BIGGEST CHALLENGE: Keeping it organized!

Design Surprises

The butterflies on the ceiling in Ripley's room, and hanging lots of small, simple art together, gallery style, for a more interesting look.

THE PLAYROOM IS . . . Organic, fun, ever changing.

RIPLEY'S ROOM IS . . . French, girlie, pink.

TANNER'S ROOM IS . . . Native American, earthy, safari.

Get the Look

PLAYROOM: I think a playroom needs to be kid-friendly and not too precious. We filled ours with tons of wooden toys that the kids actually want to play with (Camden Rose is a must!). And for an affordable and still-modern touch, I like mixing in IKEA pieces with the rest of the room. For softness, I added tablecloths and sheepskins, which add comfort to the room (we're constantly hanging out on the plush rug). The process of hanging the kids' art has been especially fun—not only does it add pops of color, it also makes them feel so good. Tanner loves hanging his own artwork now!

RIPLEY'S ROOM: Kids' rooms are a great place to mix high and low (like an expensive rug and more-affordable framed art). My goal was to create a room that was white and bright, like a French dollhouse, but I ended up going a little pink-crazy as soon as I found out I was having a girl. But I stuck with my French theme by picking out a more classic crib and changing table from Bonton, and adding a butterfly creation, which then gave me the idea to add the bird and butterfly posters, as well as the framed bugs and butterflies from my sister Saree's Evolution.

TANNER'S ROOM: Tanner's room is really all about the teepee, which I found on Amazon! With the addition of a neon dream catcher, the room really came to life. I love how I

was able to add simple pops of color to the white-and-cream backdrop with the stuffed-animal trophies and arrows.

Resources

PLAYROOM (seen on pages 38 and 39)

★ Lawrence of La Brea rug
★ Geronimo Balloon-Troopers balloons
★ Great Plains teepee from Amazon
★ Kimmel Kids dream catcher
★ FAO Schwarz elephant
★ Custom-built sliding door console
★ Woven bins available through Jenni Kayne stores
★ Confetti System garland
★ Lost and Found xylophone

RIPLEY'S ROOM

★ Bonton changing table and crib bedding
★ Wendy Addison wall hanging
★ Blanc D'Ivoire chandelier
★ Framed Hermès scarf
★ Smallable framed print and rocking sheep
★ Vintage settee
★ Bloom & Plume butterfly installation

TANNER'S ROOM

★ Oeuf Sparrow Crib
★ Rug Company rug
★ Roost pouf, available through Jenni Kayne stores
★ Smallable deer nightlight
★ Cavern wallpaper on the back of shelving unit

Athena CALDERONE

INTERIOR DESIGNER

Son Jivan, photographed at nine years old
Brooklyn, New York

This Brooklyn-based interior designer and founder of design blog EyeSwoon, has devoted her professional and personal life to creating modern, minimalist spaces with just the right amount of warmth and romance. Calderone has managed to carve out a place for herself as a go-to designer for chic children's spaces (she reinterprets high-end modern interiors for the under-ten set). An interior designer by trade, her innate sense of style has also made her a natural muse for designer friends like Dolce & Gabbana, who created her wedding dress, and fellow Glow mama Jennifer Fisher. Rounding out her tight-knit trio is husband Victor (he's a DJ who has collaborated with Madonna and Beyoncé) and surf-obsessed son Jivan.

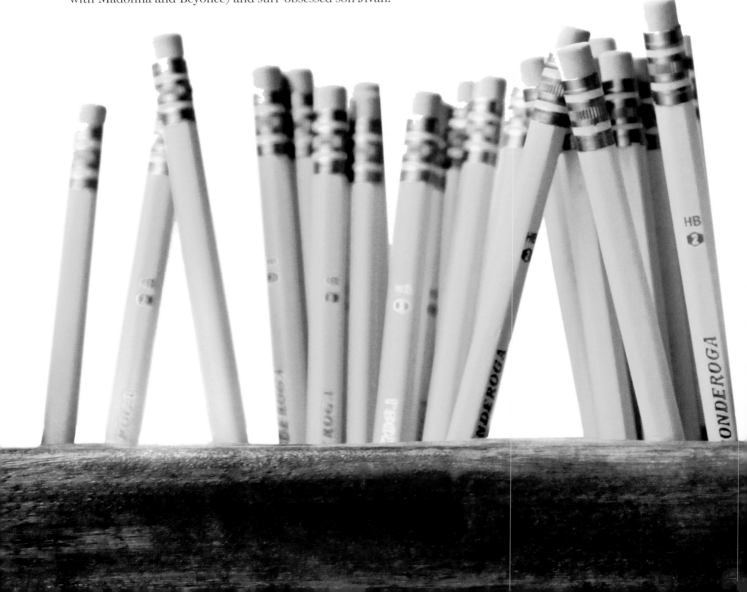

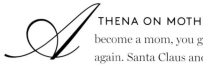**THENA ON MOTHERHOOD:** When you become a mom, you get to believe in magic again. Santa Claus and the excitement of Christmas morning, playing hide-and-seek, running around barefoot on the grass, having water-balloon fights, getting messy and not caring, going sledding and having snowball fights, dancing and spinning around until you fall on the floor in a ball of dizzy laughter. Having a child has helped me let go!

HARDEST PART: I wish I was better at not reacting immediately to frustrating moments, at letting go of the "to-do list," and being fully present when I'm with Jivan.

FAVORITE PART OF THE DAY: Every night at bedtime all three of us climb up the ladder of Jivan's bed. We end by piling on top of each other before Jivan goes to sleep.

ROOM STYLE: *The Modern Mix*
With its graphic wall art, clever built-ins, and boyishly cool touches, this surf-inspired space epitomizes Brooklyn chic.

PHILOSOPHY: I love to include Jivan in the design process. He already has such a trained eye and has been on construction and job sites since he was tiny. Visual beauty is my passion, and it's so important for him to see and understand what inspires Mommy. I love hearing his opinion and always ask for his design feedback.

Inspiration

As Jivan was getting older and beginning to develop a stronger sense of self, I wanted his room to reflect his current interests—skating and surfing—while still feeling playful, bold, and energetic, like his personality. The outcome is a space Jivan enjoys being in, creating in, and one he can grow into.

THE MIX: Many of the pieces were recycled from our prior apartment and his "younger" room, like the loft bed, which I designed. The vintage mid-century modern Sputnik light fixture has always found a place in our homes, and with the high ceilings of Jivan's room, it seemed to work perfectly for the space, adding sophistication and whimsy. It also gave the room a grown-up feel, while still being playful (it reminds Jivan of fireworks). Adding something vintage and special makes him feel proud to have a "grown-up" piece in his room.

STARTING POINT: The bold and graphic wall mural was the starting point. Jivan chose the graphite and yellow colors. Every time people enter the room, they instantly respond to this strong feature—it's the room's anchor!

Save & Splurge

Save: The rug is IKEA, and Jivan's desk is from West Elm. I also chose to manipulate and alter many beloved pieces that we already had: A white Cappellini chair that I used for my desk in our last apartment was sprayed the same yellow as the wall graphic and used as Jivan's desk chair; I took orange coat hooks and had them spray-painted the same turquoise as Jivan's Sanskrit name; and I took a large series of colorful, lacquered "jellybean" art that used to hang in our living room and hung them over Jivan's bed (I picked four of the brightest colors). I love reusing and repurposing items for new uses—it's creative to find new homes for old pieces.
Splurge: We spent the most on hiring an artist, Kim from Kamp Studios, to work on the large graphic of Jivan's name in Sanskrit, which means "to give life" (Jivan chose the color, "Surf Blue"). The custom linen roman shades were also a bit of a splurge.

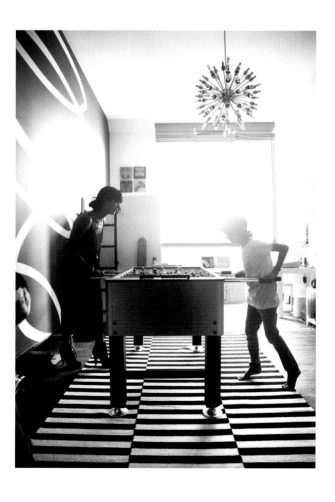

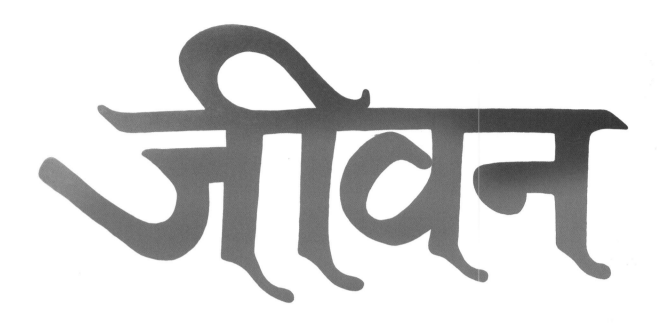

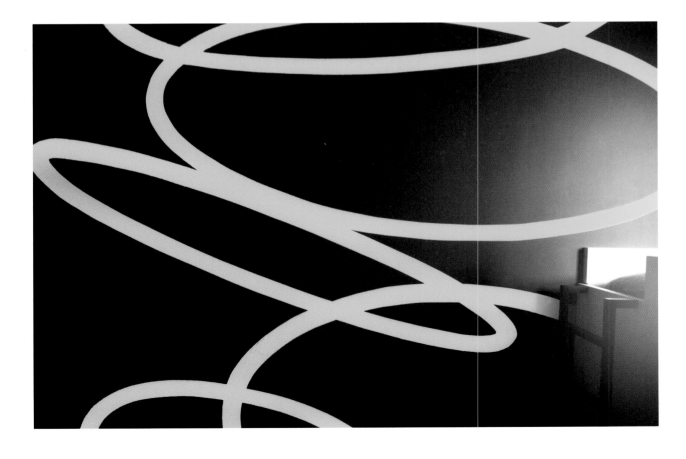

HOMEMADE TOUCHES: The tape artwork was something Jivan and I created together—we purchased an array of bold-colored gaffer and electrical tape and covered a canvas with alternating colors and varying thicknesses. Jivan chose the colors and the order we applied the colors. It's so important for children to feel involved in creating their surroundings—it gives them a sense of pride and connectedness to their space. We also framed some of the watercolor "splatter" artwork Jivan made in school in white gallery frames.

PERSONAL TOUCHES: The *puja*, a place for him to keep things that are sacred to him—photos, artwork, mementos. Jivan has had it in his room since he was three. There are many rocks and shells we have collected together from trips and various items that hold special memories.

BIGGEST CHALLENGE: Spatial planning: The room is large, yet long and narrow, so creating certain "zones" (play, homework, toy storage, sleeping) took some creativity to find an ideal layout.

Design Surprises

I had purchased a wooden mold on eBay, and I never quite knew what to use it for. When Jivan chose yellow for his room, and with the sudden need for lots of pencils for homework, I chose to fill this rustic wooden object with lots of utilitarian basic yellow number-two pencils. It's a great art installation that's also useful. I also love juxtaposing punchy bright colors against either dark or light walls. You see this in many areas within the room—from the wall graphics to the yellow desk chair and the vertical coat hooks.

ROOM DÉCOR IN THREE WORDS: Bold, playful, graphic

JIVAN'S ROOM IS . . . The space really represents Jivan growing up and becoming a boy, rather than a preschooler. The ritual of using the foosball table every night before bed speaks to his coordination and is an engaging activity the whole family enjoys—it continues to create memories for us all.

Get the Look

- ★ Vintage chandelier for a bit of glamour
- ★ Dark walls to add edge
- ★ Pops of bold color to brighten things up
- ★ Jivan's framed artwork to add personality and pride

Resources

- ★ Athena-designed bunk bed, made by a local furniture maker
- ★ IKEA striped rug
- ★ Vintage mid-century modern Sputnik chandelier purchased more than a decade ago from Lost City Arts (the first major piece Athena and her husband, Victor, bought together as a couple)
- ★ West Elm bedding
- ★ West Elm parsons desk

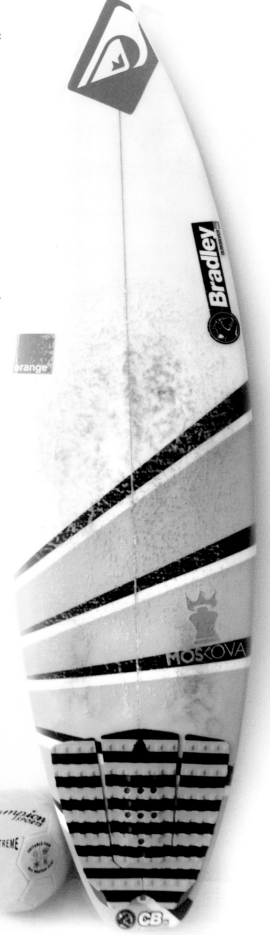

Laura PORETZKY-GARCIA

CREATIVE DIRECTOR & COFOUNDER OF ÉTÉ

Daughter Georgiana ("Gigi"),
photographed at fifteen months old
New York, New York

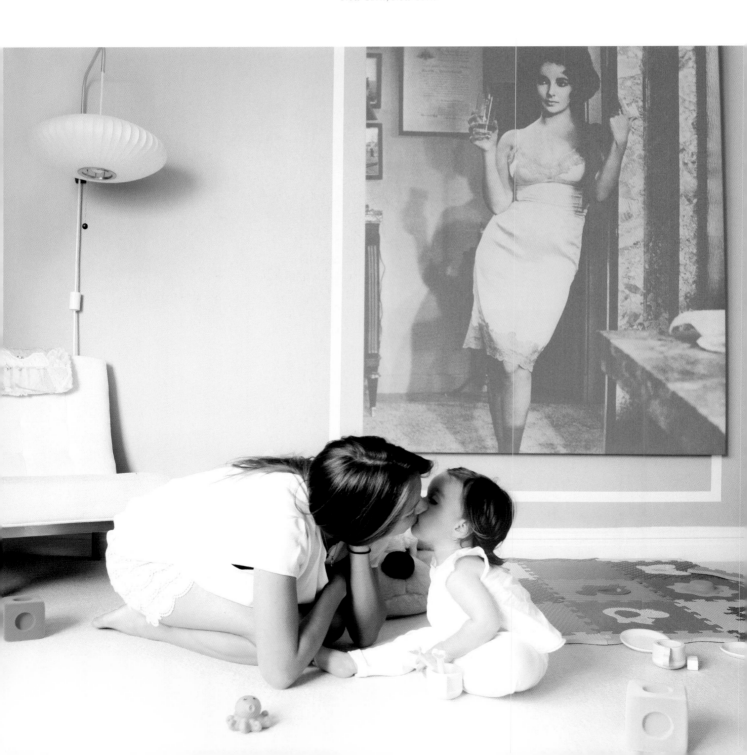

This French-Brazilian designer gained instant success in 2004 with her ready-to-wear line Abaeté. The collection was scooped up by Bergdorf Goodman and Intermix, and eventually turned into a lucrative collaboration with Payless. After becoming a mom, Garcia shifted her focus to freelance work so she could spend more time with her daughter, Georgiana. Now she's back in the fashion game with her retro-inspired swimwear line, Été. She and her musician husband, Diego, raise their trilingual baby in an elegant space sprinkled with art, books stacked floor-to-ceiling, and family photos. When they're not on tour with Diego, mother and child explore the city to-gether—frequenting the very same spots that Laura, who grew up just a few blocks away, treasured as a kid.

LAURA ON MOTHERHOOD: A mom I have always looked up to is my own mother. She's always made an effort to be a friend. I can tell her everything, and she really is my best friend. I hope I will be that for Gigi one day.

HARDEST PART: I was such a routine person before she was born—I had a time to do everything. Then she came along, and I worked so hard to put her on a routine. All of a sudden, though, I come second, and my life revolves around her.

ROOM STYLE: *Minimalist Meets Luxe*
The combination of cool gray walls, sophisticated art, and vintage touches prove that chic simplicity works at any age.

Inspiration

The design inspiration was based around what the rest of the apartment looked like—I didn't want my daughter's room to stick out like a sore thumb. Our aesthetic is a little bit glam, mixed with some seventies inspiration. I love gray for the walls because it doesn't scream "girl," but it's still soft and feminine.

Save & Splurge

Save: I think you can always save on storage—whatever you end up getting will look cute, as long as it's filled with all of their adorable toys.
Splurge: I really think that getting a nice crib is important. They spend so much time in there, and later on it can be handed down to the next child.

Design Surprises

The white carpet actually doesn't show much, believe it or not. You can't imagine how many times she's thrown up on it. Since we are only in this apartment temporarily, I added some faux molding to the gray walls to create a graphic effect. I think it really works.

MOST CHALLENGING: Keeping it cool and simple, while still girly.

GEORGIANA'S ROOM IS . . . Soothing, calm, clean, and modern.

Get the Look

I mixed bold, grown-up artwork with girly yet minimal neutrals and vintage elements. By adding faux molding for graphic effect and keeping the color just in the art, the room feels a bit unexpected.

Resources

★ Vintage chair
★ Design Within Reach sconce
★ "Grey Ember" wall paint by Benjamin Moore
★ Russell Young print

Jeanann WILLIAMS

Daughter Ruby, photographed at three years old
Montauk, New York

Before landing at True Religion, Jeanann Williams worked her magic on brands like Alexander Wang and Victoria's Secret while at powerhouse agency KCD. With years of fashion experience under her belt, she's now flexing her styling muscles working with, among others, actress (and aunt to daughter, Ruby) Naomi Watts. With her own laid-back style and effortless approach to motherhood, Williams embodies the understated charm inherent in the East End town she calls home. Beach chic meets cool sophistication at her rustic modern Montauk house. The young mom has passed her easygoing sensibility on to her daughter, already a world traveler; Ruby's eclectic bedroom reflects her globe-trotting upbringing—France, Ibiza, and Australia all before her second birthday.

JEANANN ON MOTHERHOOD: I didn't find out beforehand that I was having a girl. It's the biggest surprise life can give you. It's one of those important lessons to learn as you enter parenthood—there are tons of surprises and things you can't control.

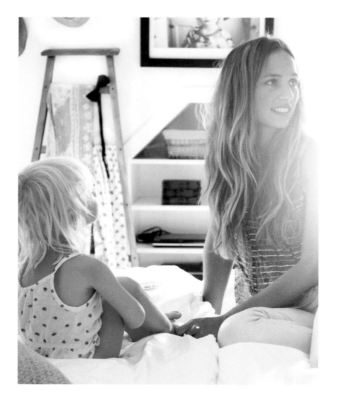

HARDEST PART: I wish I could spend my days in Ruby's world. I don't want to miss a thing.

ROOM STYLE: *Bohemian Chic*
The quintessential laid-back beach vibe comes to life in this effortlessly put-together space defined by simple touches: Restoration Hardware bed, Anthropologie pillows, Wisteria rug, and a vintage hand-me-down desk.

BIGGEST CHALLENGE: A child's room has endless possibilities, which can seem challenging, but you can really let yourself go wild and have fun with it. The most important thing was ensuring that the space inspired creativity. Ruby's room continues to evolve—as she grows, the room begins to tell a story all its own.

RUBY'S ROOM IS . . . Bohemian, whimsical, princess-approved.

Get the Look

Using a feminine color palette was important. Vintage touches give it that lived-and-loved feeling, while creating a cohesive feel with the rest of the home. Mixing prints, colors, and fabrics gives it a beachy, bohemian vibe.

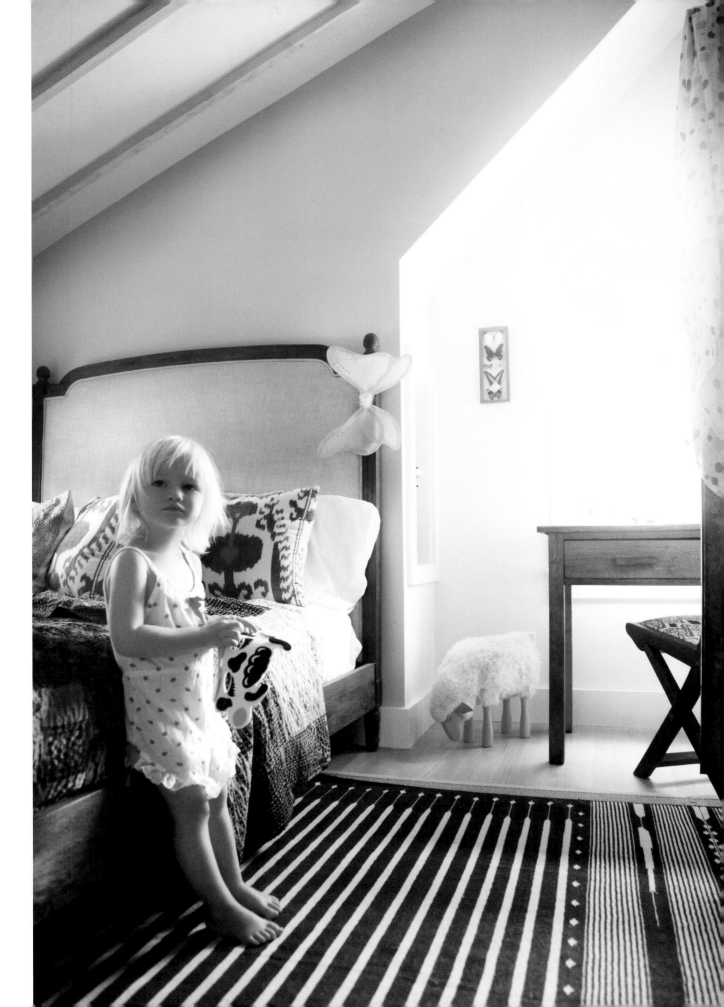

Jade BERREAU

ARTIST

Daughter Secret,
photographed at four years old
Brooklyn, New York

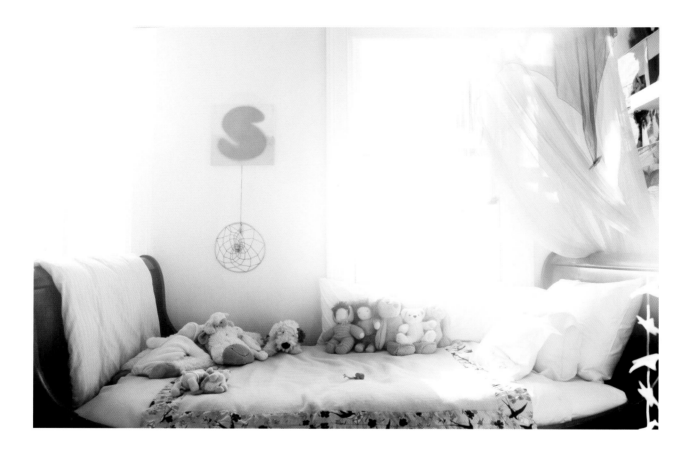

The second you step into Jade Berreau's Brooklyn brownstone, a feeling of calm washes over you. The vibrating, sometimes maddening buzz of New York melts away. In its place is the sound of old jazz records wafting through the light-filled space. The Paris-born, Manhattan-raised artist and photo editor lives with her daughter, Secret (whose father is the late artist Dash Snow), in a home that is steeped in warmth and affection. Snow's spirit is felt at every turn, with family photos and pieces of his artwork scattered throughout the three floors. Not surprisingly, Secret's room—filled with plush stuffed animals, draped silk, and whimsical music boxes—is the most magical part of the house.

JADE ON MOTHERHOOD: There's a piece of advice I heard when I was twelve years old, and it always made sense to me: Communicate with your child. Explain things rather than saying "because I say so."

HARDEST PART: Consistency. I try my best to make sure that I make one-on-one time with Secret.

BEST PART: Every time I look at her, I feel a sense of pride. It's mind-blowing to have been a part of creating a life.

ROOM STYLE: *Eclectic Cool*
Filled with family heirlooms, draped silk, and vintage music boxes, this girlishly whimsical space is the perfect mix of magical and meaningful.

Inspiration

She was three when we moved in, and it was going to be her first real bedroom, so I wanted it to be warm, inviting, and fun.

STARTING POINT: The bed was the starting point. It's a family heirloom that began with my great-grandfather—it was mine when I was younger, too.

PERSONAL TOUCHES: I put together a wall of family photos (shown at right) over Secret's bed. The one of Secret and me covered in paint was taken by my mom one summer in Sag Harbor. I want to keep adding to this collection.

Save & Splurge

Save: I've kept it pretty simple—I had a basic bookshelf built and stacked it with her toys and books.
Splurge: If I were to splurge, it would be on bedding!

HOMEMADE TOUCHES: She was once given about a dozen beautiful, handmade small animals. I found them too special to play with and possibly lose, so I strung them on fishing string, and they now float below the ceiling all in a row. She loves it!

THE LITTLE MOMENTS: I always enjoy tidying her room and putting away all the tiny details—it calms me, and she loves to help.

SECRET'S ROOM IS . . . Pink, tranquil, and inviting.

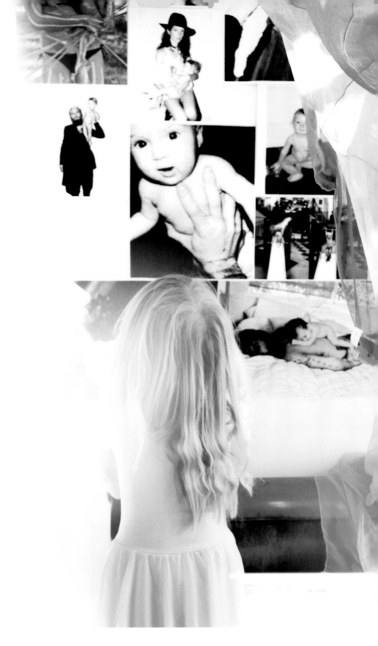

Get the Look

I started off with all of the great hand-me-downs I've been given, and then I splashed the room with all of Secret's toys. Great bedding, a good lamp for atmosphere, and beautiful curtains pulled it all together. Still, it's always a work in progress! That's the fun of it.

Resources

- ★ Vintage bed
- ★ Sarah's Silks canopy
- ★ Custom shelves

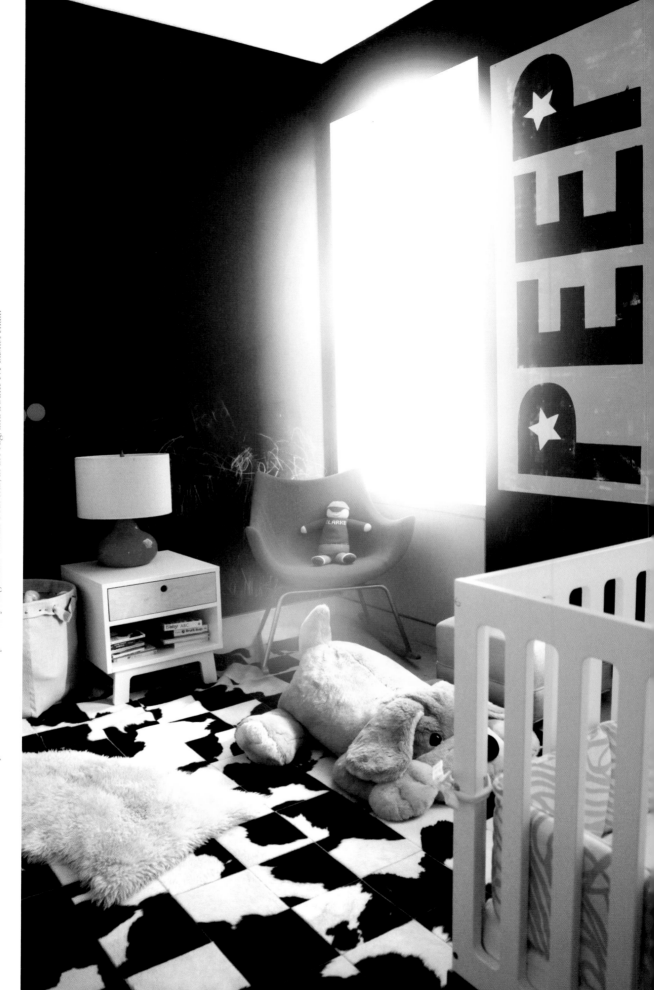

RIGHT: Ferebee Taube created a mostly black-and-white nursery for her youngest son with an Oeuf crib, aPure rug, and a Suite NY basket chair.

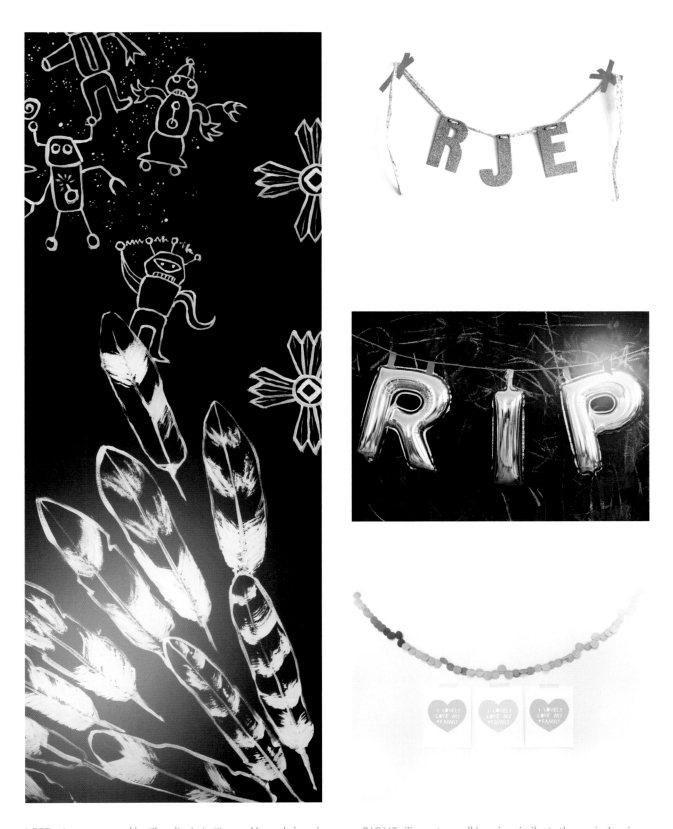

LEFT: A custom mural by Clamdiggin in Simone Harouche's son's nursery. RIGHT: To create a wall hanging similar to the one in Jenni Kayne's daughter's room (shown at top), 1) cut out letters using paper or fabric, 2) choose your ribbon, and 3) select tape (optional: stencils to ensure that the letters look uniform). Jenni took the letters, created by artist Wendy Addison, and attached them to $10 floral ribbon from Olive Manna. Then she used $4 neon-pink tape from Etsy to place it above daughter Ripley's changing table. The letter balloons from Ripley's birthday party (middle) now serve as permanent decor on the playroom wall. Jessie Randall chose a felt garland and pastel prints from Etsy for her twins' bedroom (bottom).

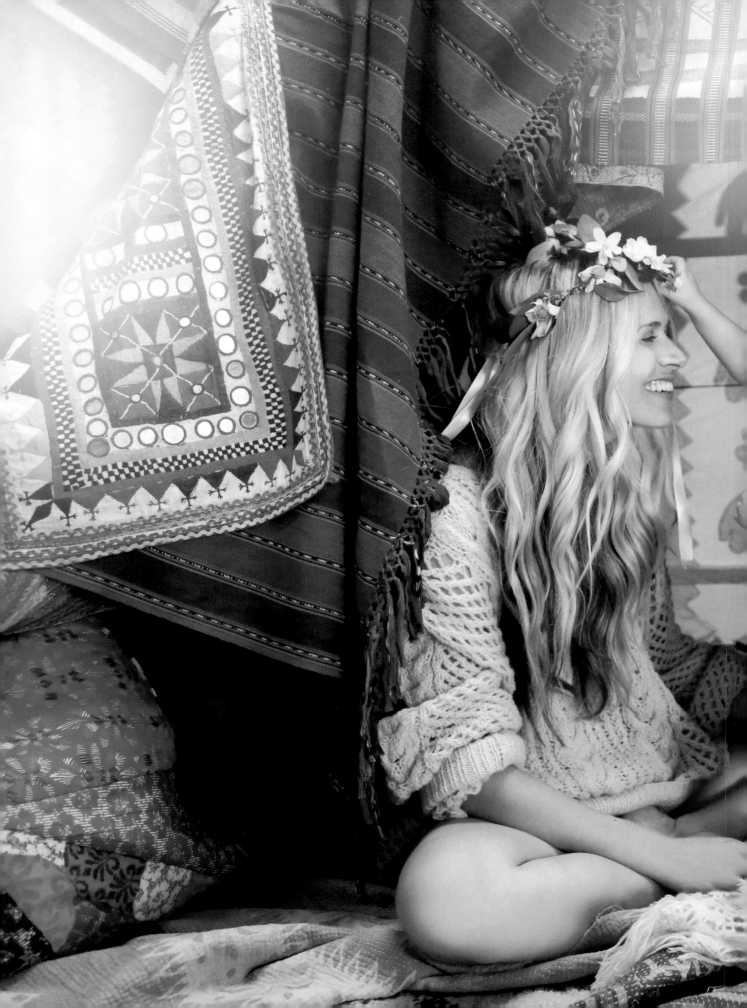

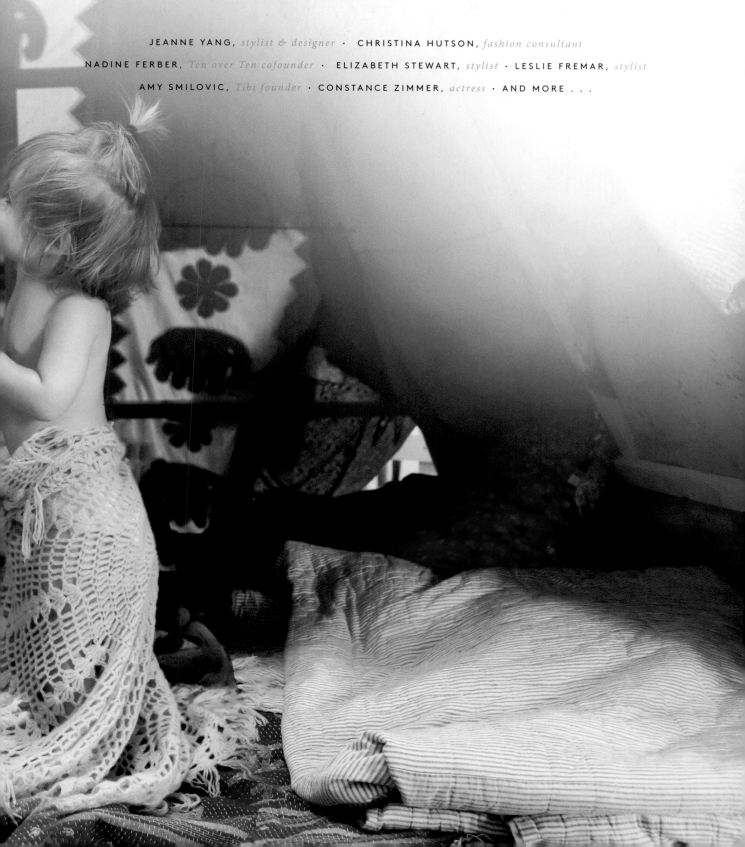

CHAPTER THREE

In the Moment

JEANNE YANG, *stylist & designer* · CHRISTINA HUTSON, *fashion consultant*

NADINE FERBER, *Ten over Ten cofounder* · ELIZABETH STEWART, *stylist* · LESLIE FREMAR, *stylist*

AMY SMILOVIC, *Tibi founder* · CONSTANCE ZIMMER, *actress* · AND MORE . . .

*A*s a mom of three boys, including twins, Julie Bowen (pictured on page 142) would seem to know a thing or two about creating balance. But the actress admits that being a mom is "pure joy and pure challenge all the time." During rare moments of calm, Bowen takes a "mental picture to file away," and tells herself, "This is good. This is what it's all about. It will never be better than this moment."

One of the reasons Kelly and I decided to create The Glow was to explore this concept of balance—was it possible, and if so, how could we achieve it? What we found is that there's no one-size-fits-all answer. Bottom line: Making time to devote your whole heart to multiple roles—individual, partner, and mother—can feel overwhelming at times. Jemima Kirke, mom of two, artist, and actress, explains, "In order of importance: 1. Self, 2. Marriage, 3. Child. Of course all are important, but neglecting the one before is a disservice to the one after." In a similar vein, makeup artist Pati Dubroff lives by this common sense rule: "Just like in the safety instructions you're given when flying, it's important to first give yourself the life vest and oxygen before helping others."

In this chapter we explore the beautiful yet complex journey of the working mother—from stylist Jeanann Williams's nanny-envy to the nightly mother-daughter routine actress Constance Zimmer swears by. These multitasking moms reveal their struggles and the secrets to maintaining their most meaningful relationships without losing themselves along the way.

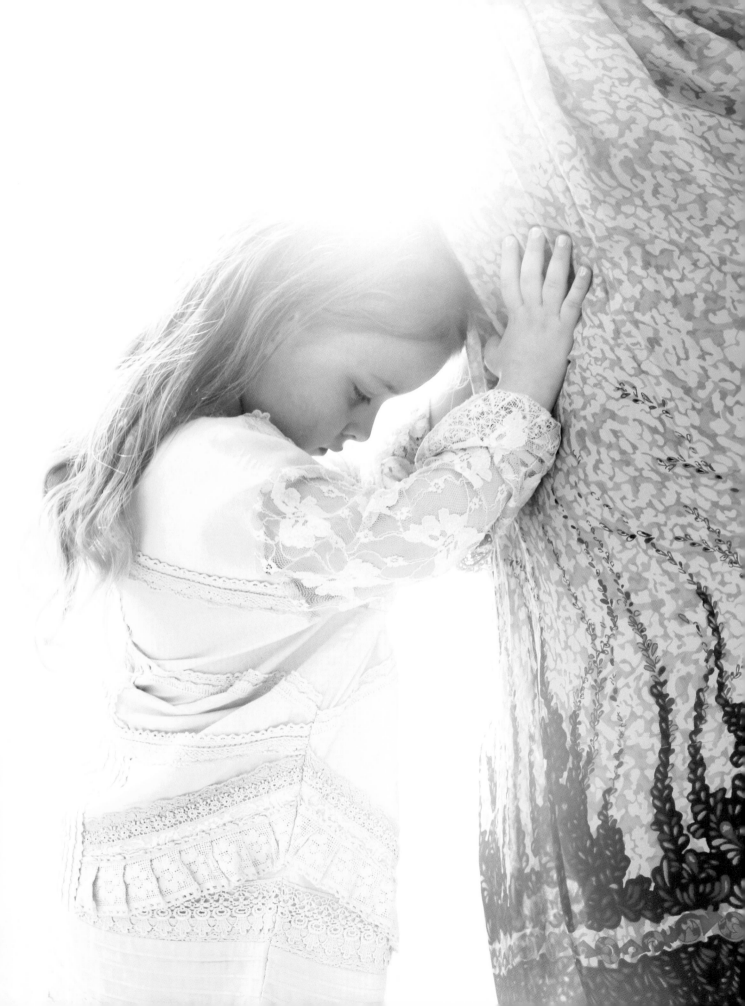

"*The best moment of my life
was when my ladies were born,
and it's only gotten better.*"

—*Jeanne Yang,* STYLIST & DESIGNER

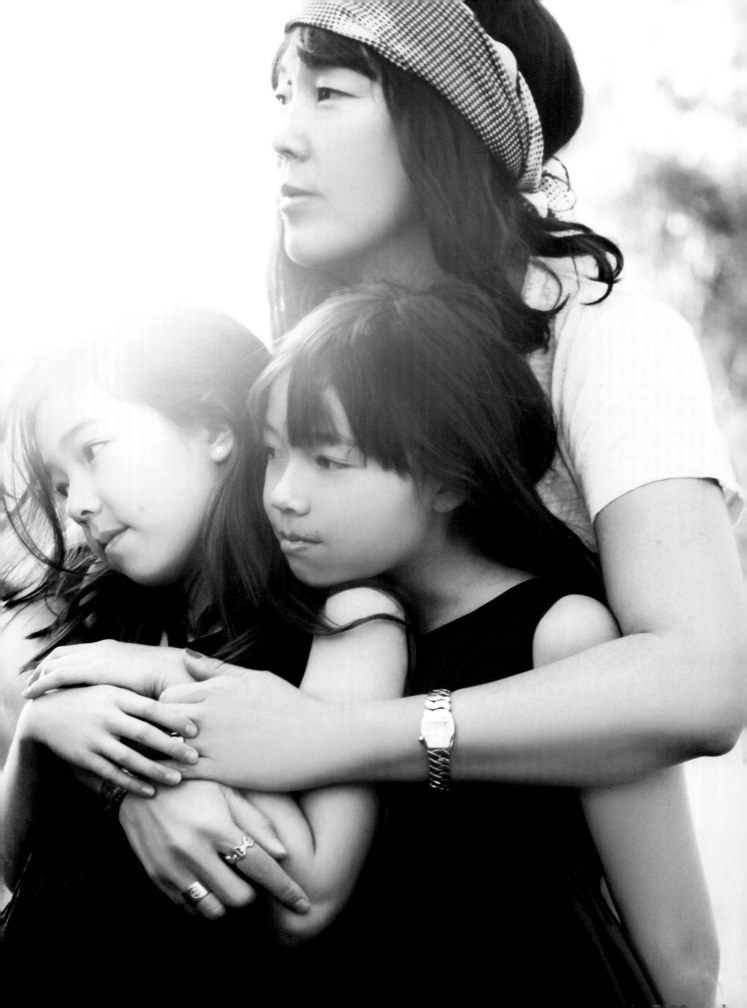

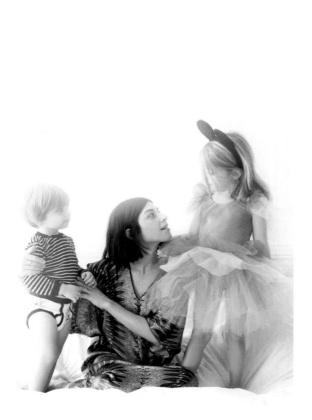

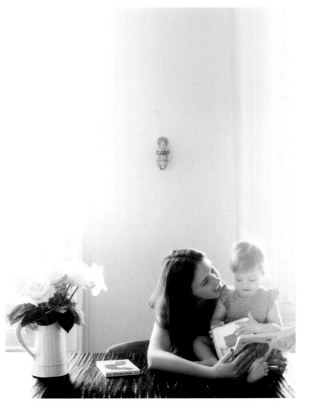

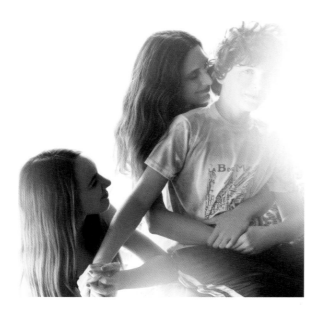

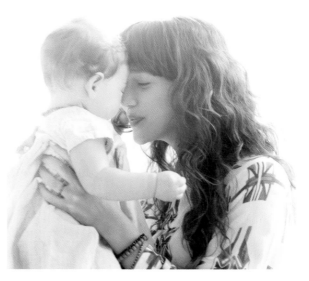

CLOCKWISE FROM TOP LEFT: Christina Hutson with Lowe and Valentine; Nadine Ferber with Zoe Lee; Zoë Buckman with Cleo; Elizabeth Stewart with Ben and Ivy.

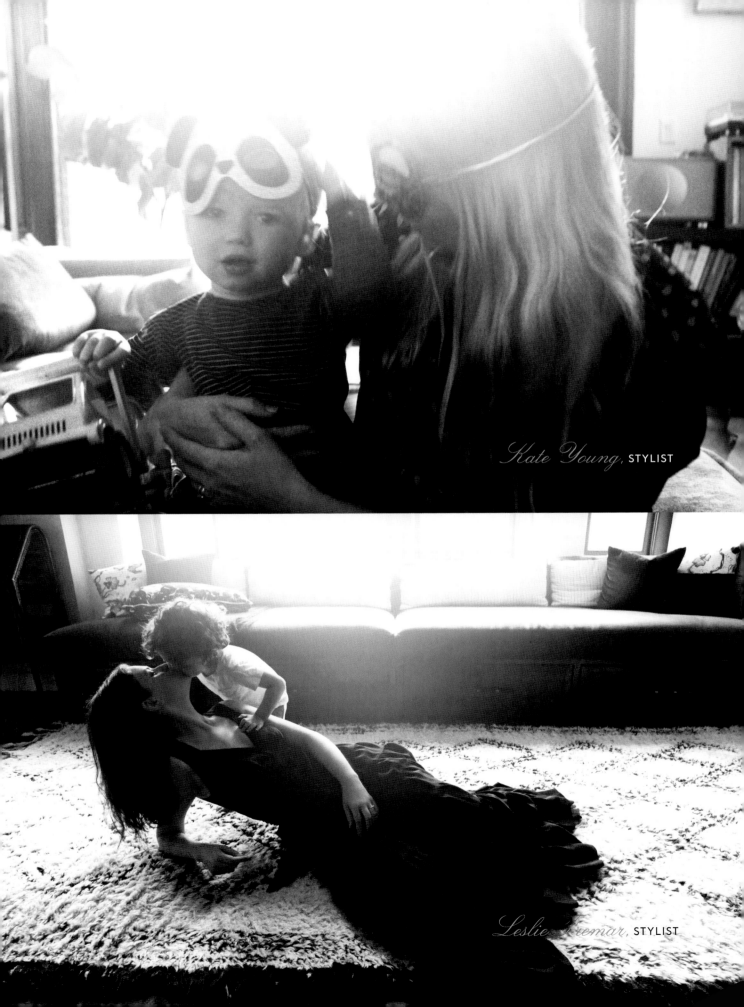

Kate Young, STYLIST

Leslie Fremar, STYLIST

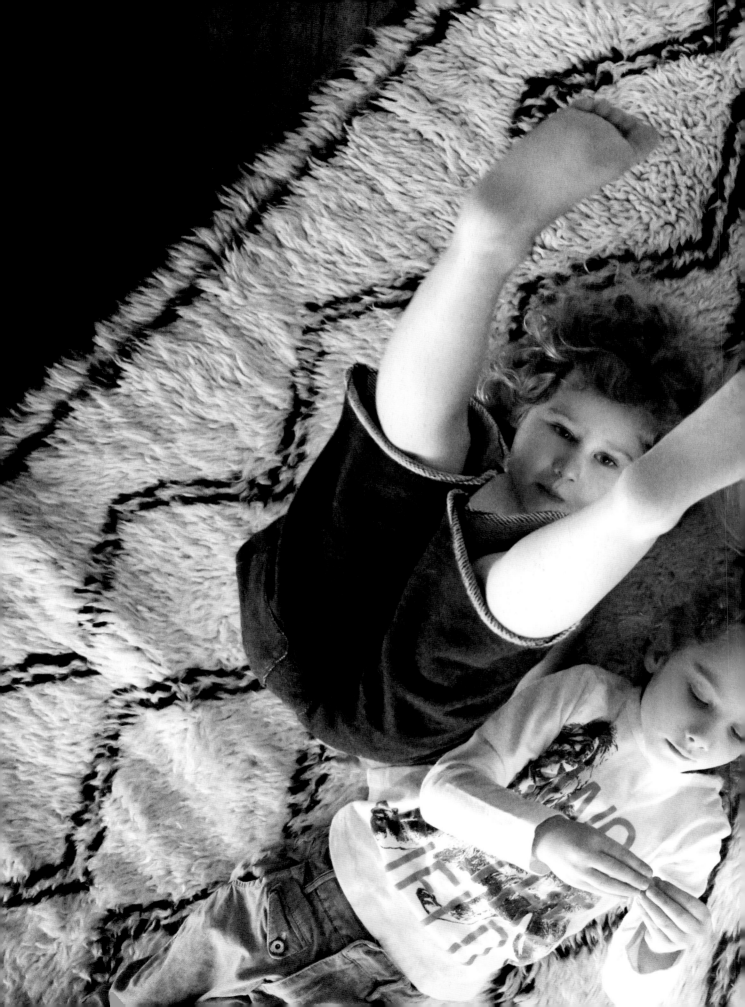

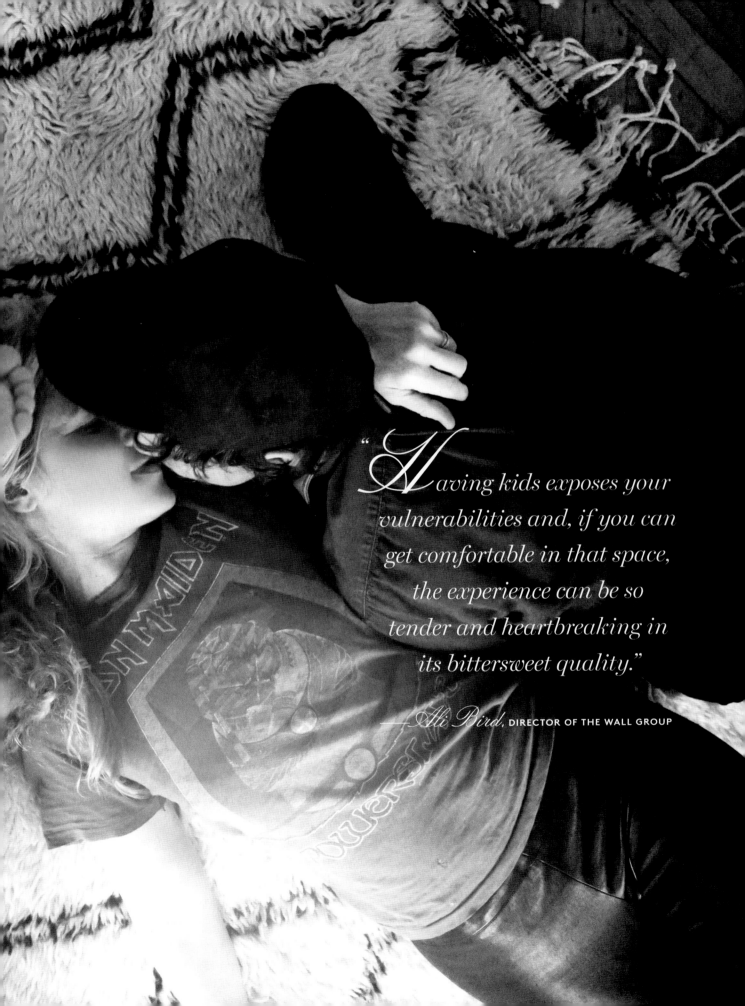

"*Having kids exposes your vulnerabilities and, if you can get comfortable in that space, the experience can be so tender and heartbreaking in its bittersweet quality.*"

—*Ali Bird*, **DIRECTOR OF THE WALL GROUP**

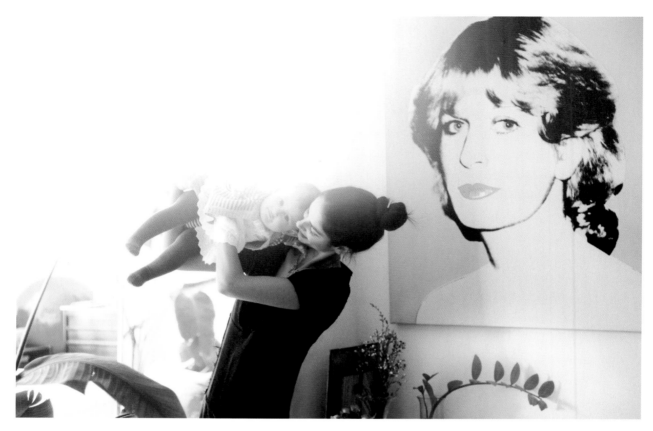

ABOVE: "My husband and I are very open about our feelings towards each other, and hearing that you are loved and appreciated before you collapse into bed makes you realize that all is good."—*Ana Lerario-Geller* BELOW: "Acceptance, laughter, and self-reflection are my secrets to a long-lasting relationship."—*Jeanine Lobell*

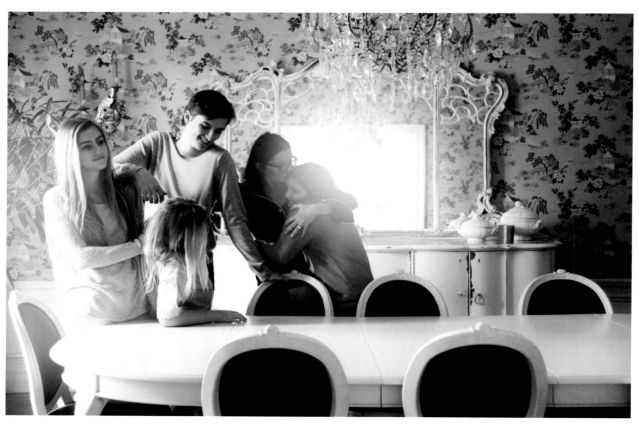

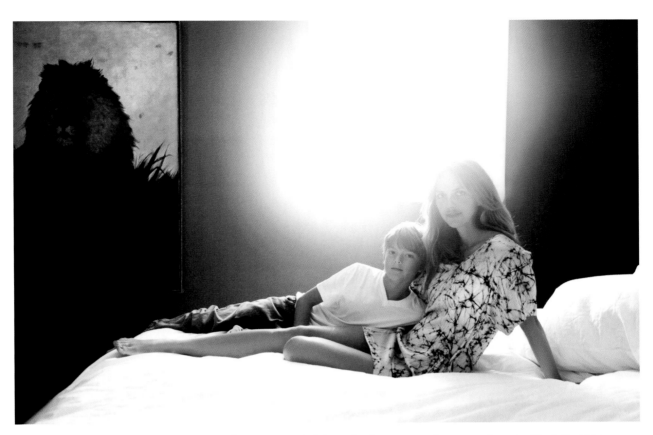

ABOVE: "Being with my husband in situations where we are not judging each other as parents is very, very important!"—*Leilani Bishop*
BELOW: "My advice for balancing motherhood and marriage: Make sure you shower. It's important to still care about yourself and your appearance."—*Amy Smilovic*

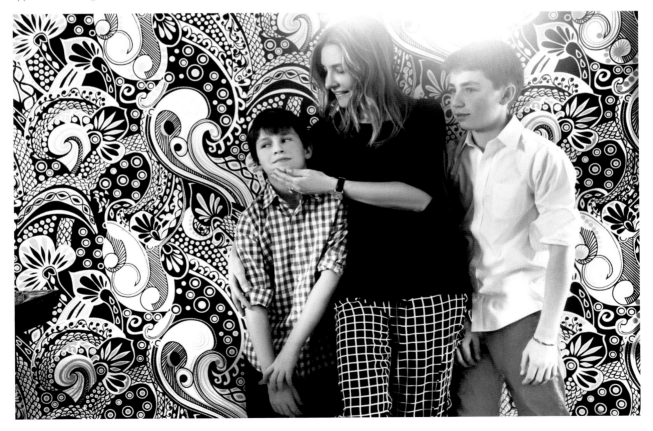

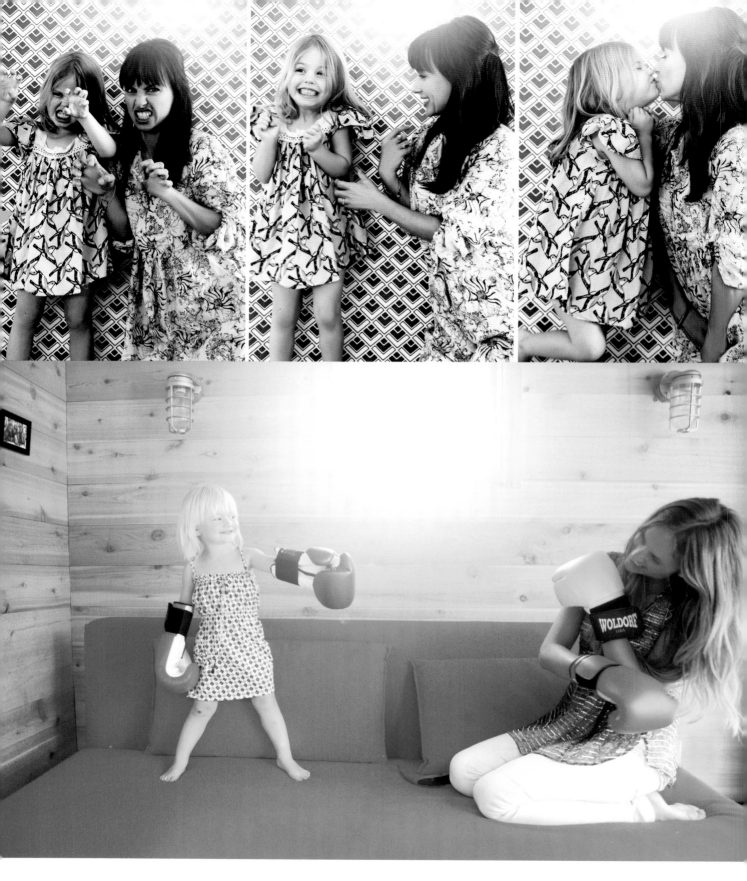

ABOVE: "Every night after we read books, we turn the lights off and talk about the day and say all the things that we are thankful for."
—*Constance Zimmer* BELOW: "I often envy our nanny—I wish I could spend my days in Ruby's world going on play dates, taking trips to the water park, watching her spin round and round in Tots and Tutus class. I don't want to miss a thing. I always wonder, how many 'firsts' does she have in a day? It's magical to be a part of that sense of discovery." —*Jeanann Williams*

IN THE MOMENT

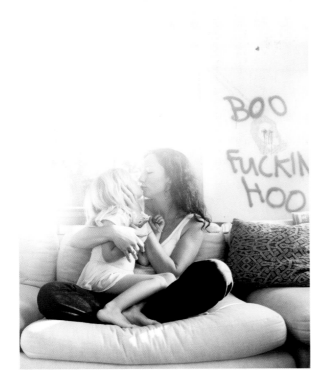

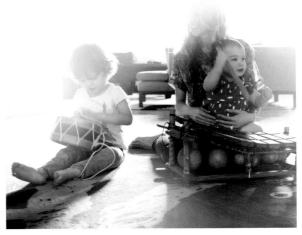

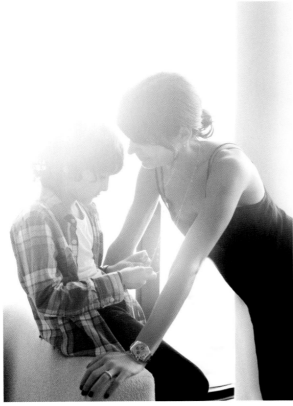

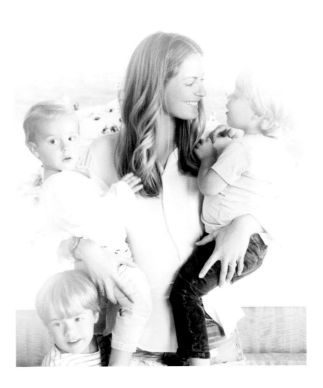

CLOCKWISE FROM TOP LEFT: Jade Berreau with Secret; Eleanor Ylvisaker with Alastair and Ella; Ferebee Taube wiht Bishop, Ford, and Clarke; Athena Calderone with Jivan

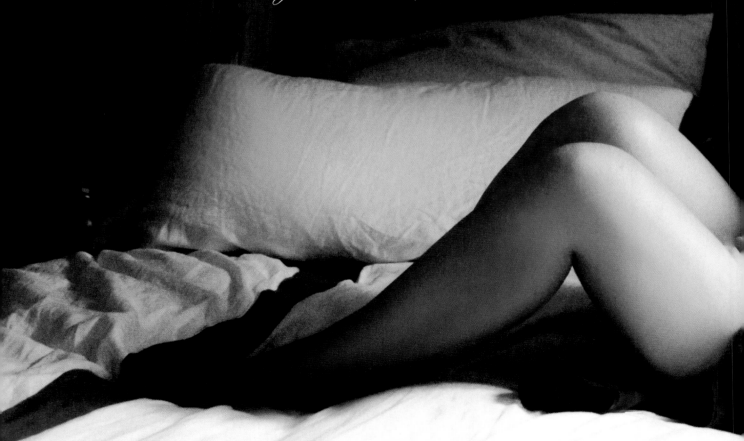

"*Since having children,
losing each other poses
a much greater threat.
There's no abandoning ship.
But it's in those challenges that
I've truly gotten to know
my husband and actually
fallen more in love with him.*"

—*Jemima Kirke*, **ARTIST & ACTRESS**

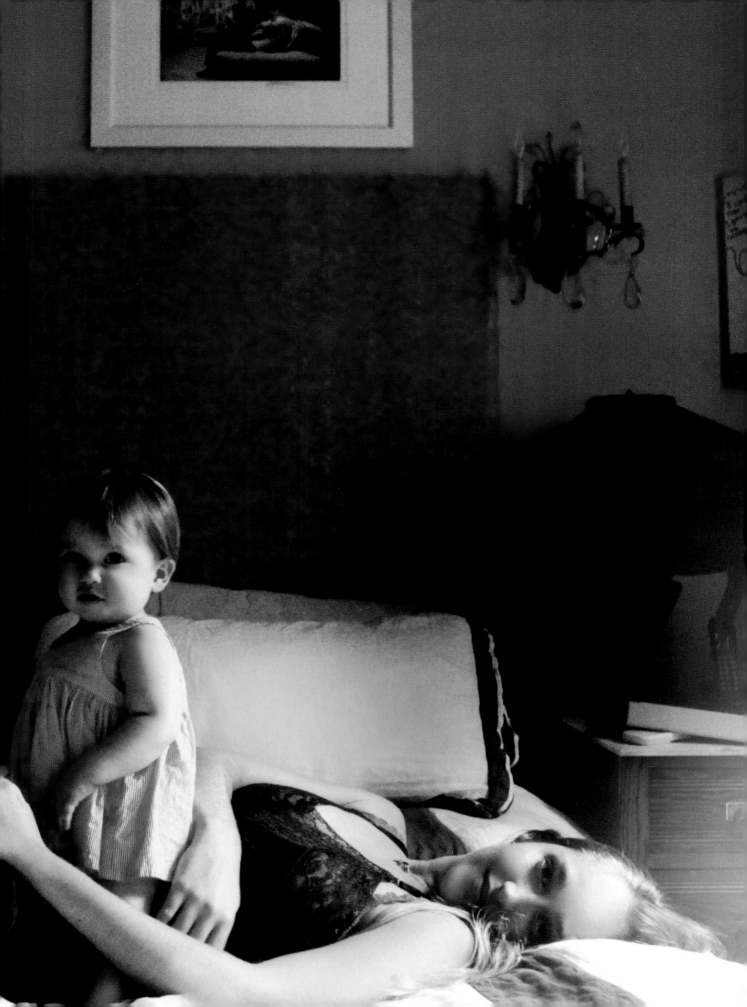

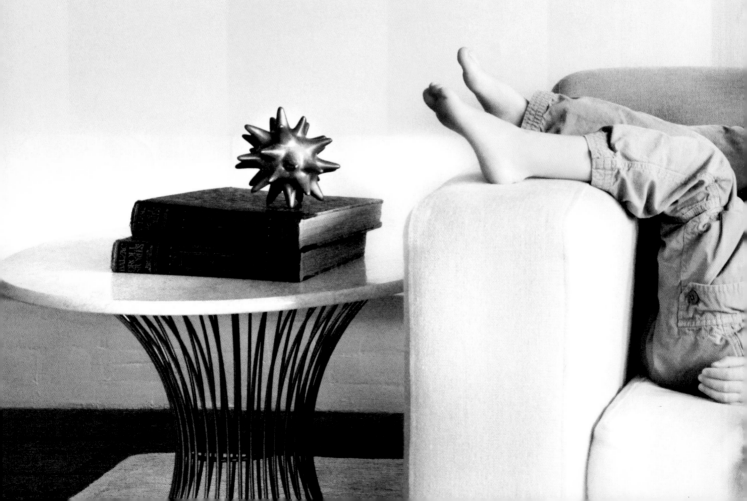

CHAPTER FOUR

Inspiring Interiors

CHRISTIANE LEMIEUX, *founder & creative director, DwellStudio*

AMY NEUNSINGER, *photographer* · CALGARY AVANSINO, *British Vogue contributing editor & health expert*

JEMMA KIDD, *beauty expert* · KATHRYN NEALE, *stylist*

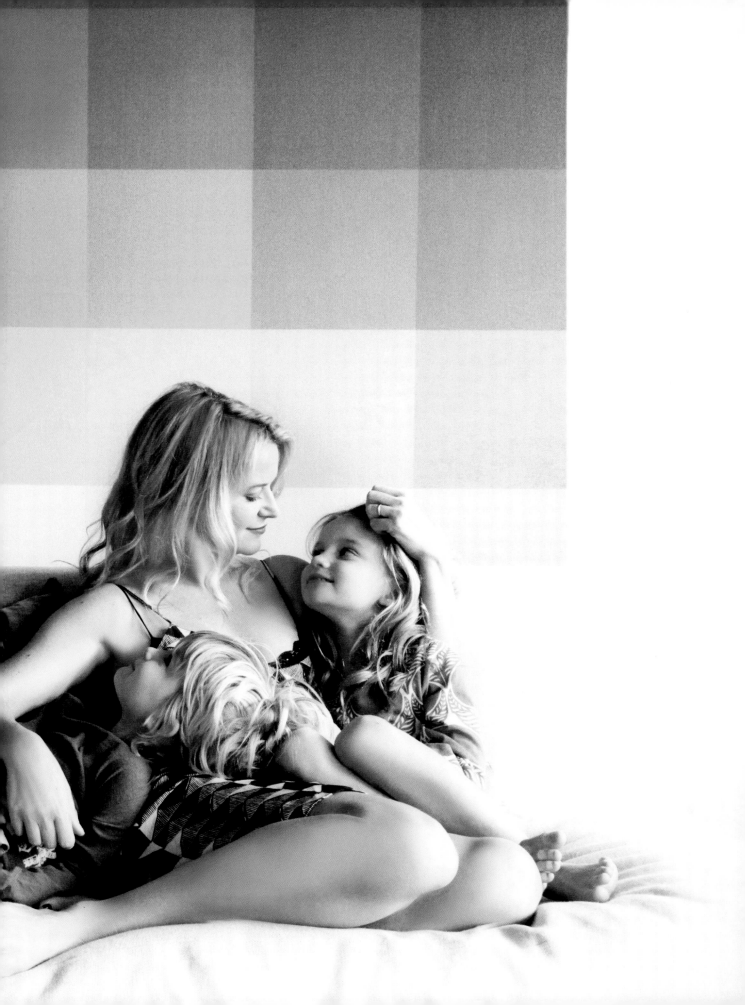

I want people to walk into my house and be surprised that there's a baby." Most moms can surely relate to artist and actress Jemima Kirke's simple wish. The desire to keep her home from looking like a "jungle gym" led Kirke to buy everything baby-related in black, beige, and white. But even this cool Brooklyn mom admits that doing so was "almost impossible."

According to British *Vogue* editor and health expert Calgary Avansino, it's all about the art of disguise. She admits that the secret to keeping her London town house looking sophisticated and highly organized is having "nearly as many baskets as we do toys. Throw everything in, and close the top."

In this chapter, we explore home décor—and how it inevitably changes once children come into the picture. In many cases, the child is incorporated into the existing design, rather than the other way around. Whitney Bromberg Hawkings, director of communications for Tom Ford (and mom of two boys under four), believes that if her children "grow up around beautiful things, they learn to appreciate and respect them."

On the opposite end of the spectrum is photographer Amy Neunsinger, who firmly believes that the chaos of family life (including a husband, a dog, and two rambunctious boys) means that everything in her Laurel Canyon home must be able to be "thrown in the wash or replaced. No one thing is more important than the people in my house."

Whether designing for a New York City loft or a sprawling English countryside estate, each of these style-minded moms describes how they've maintained the aesthetic of their sanctuaries, while making them baby-friendly, not baby-proofed.

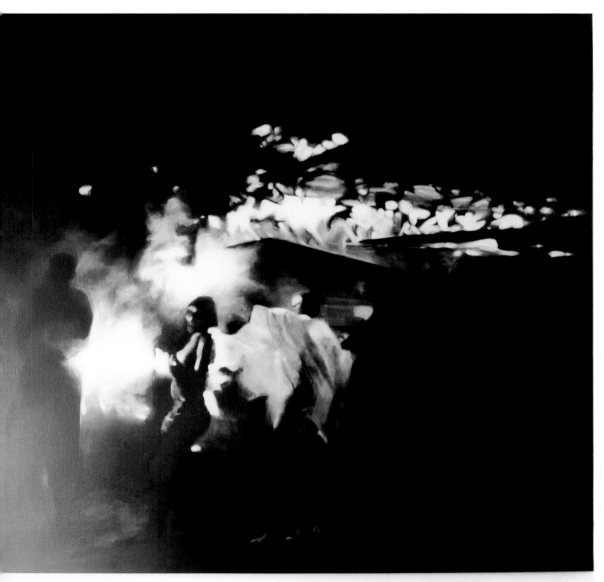
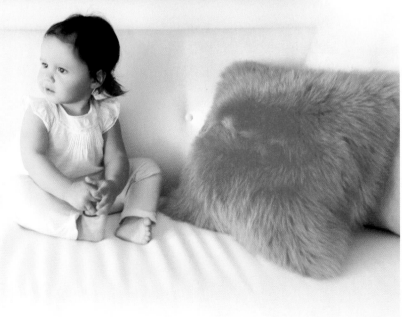

Christiane LEMIEUX

FOUNDER & CREATIVE DIRECTOR OF DWELLSTUDIO

Daughter Isabelle and son William,
photographed at five and a half and four years old, respectively
New York, New York

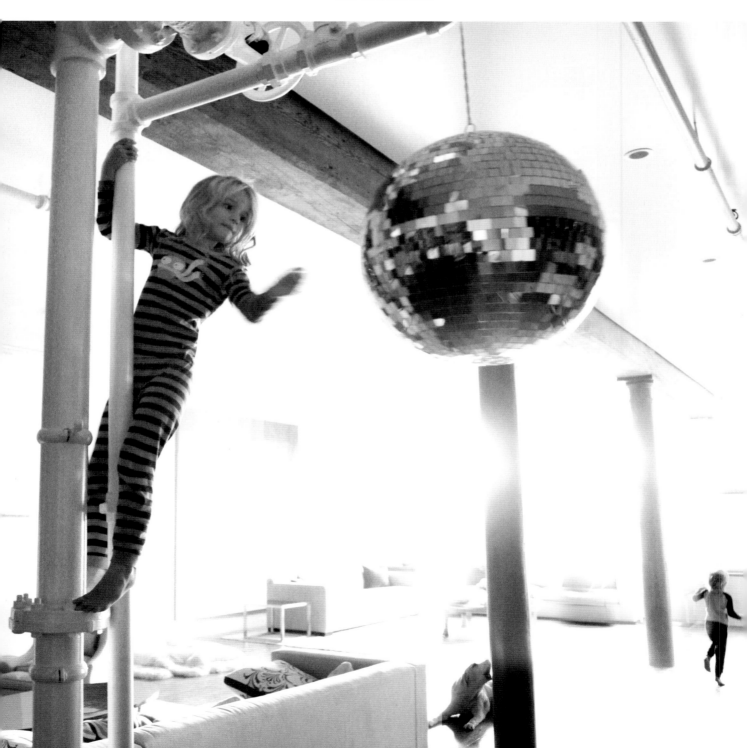

DwellStudio's founder and creative director, Christiane Lemieux, has mastered the subtle art of undone glamour, both at work and at home. Her thriving brand (husband Josh is her business partner) is best known, and much loved, for its whimsical textiles and modern décor. With its loyal following, DwellStudio has become a one-stop shop for style-minded moms—bedding, clothing, toys, even artwork. In her sprawling SoHo loft, Lemieux takes a laid-back approach to parenting: Dance parties on the antique dining table? Sure. Swinging from the disco–ball–adorned pipe in the middle of the living room? Encouraged. Raising two wildly imaginative (and polite!) kids while balancing an expanding empire, a happy marriage, and the daily school run is all in a day's work.

CHRISTIANE ON MOTHERHOOD: In the moment your child is born, your whole world changes, and it's really all about your baby. It's amazing to have a paradigm shift like that in an instant.

BEST ADVICE: My amazing sister-in-law, Karen, raised two excellent kids, and when I asked her how they turned out so well, she said it's because they ate dinner together every night. We are really trying to make that work in our family—it seems so simple, but it's not! It requires work and organization, but I can already see the benefits.

HARDEST PART: I never knew I would want to be in two places so much—the push-pull is crazy. I want to be the best mom possible and the best at my job, too. I am trying to find the balance.

HOME STYLE: *Luxe Loft*

PHILOSOPHY: No clutter. We designed our living space to be very open—this way, the kids can run around safely. I also don't get too attached to anything. With two active kids, things are going to happen.

Inspiration

Our home is a classic New York loft. I wanted to celebrate that but add luxe European details in the floors, fixtures, and cabinets. It's a bit of Amsterdam in New York.

SECRETS OF DISGUISE: I have always used matching storage bins on shelves. And get the kids' stuff out the door as soon as they are done with it. You will be happy it's gone.

THE STARTING POINT: We worked the design of the space around our dining table, which I found at the Paris flea market—it seats twenty-four! We anchored the table

with a huge chandelier that I found at Brimfield Antique Show. We have so many amazing memories of events around this table—everything is better when you are eating.

Save & Splurge

We splurged on the space and saved on the renovation by doing a lot ourselves.

Design Surprises

I painted the kitchen and the bookshelves black, and it just works.

MY HOME IS . . . Minimal, modern, luxe.

Get the Look

- ★ Mix of new and old pieces—I always go for new uphol-stery mixed with vintage finds.
- ★ Silk rugs—there is nothing more luxe than walking on silk.
- ★ Reclaimed-wood floors
- ★ Neutral, natural fabrics for upholstery
- ★ Big, dramatic art
- ★ Statement lighting fixtures—go big and bold.
- ★ Fabulous wallpaper in smaller spaces like the hall, bathrooms and closets

Resources

- ★ Robert Swain painting (seen on pages 76 and 77)
- ★ Montauk Sofa and De La Espada couches
- ★ Disco ball from Amazon
- ★ Side table from Paris flea market

Amy NEUNSINGER

PHOTOGRAPHER

Sons Jackson and August,
photographed at ten and eight years old, respectively
Los Angeles, California

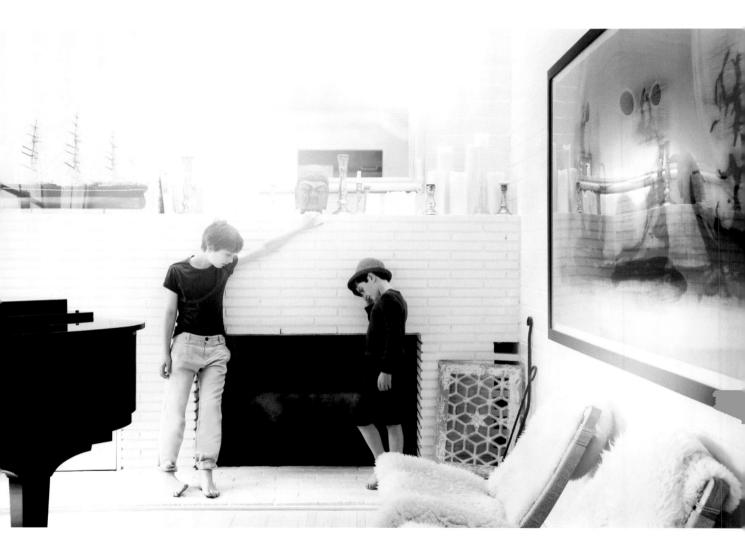

Just like her photos, which capture California's sun-drenched, laid-back lifestyle, Amy Neunsinger's home is a perfect reflection of effortless style. With its loft-like layout and mix of flea-market finds and plush Shabby Chic furnishings, it's no wonder this Laurel Canyon compound pops up constantly on Pinterest (just search "Dream House" and you'll see what we mean). Despite the mostly white décor and serene vibe, Neunsinger, mom of two boys, is happiest when chaos abounds—and lives by the motto "Everyone is welcome."

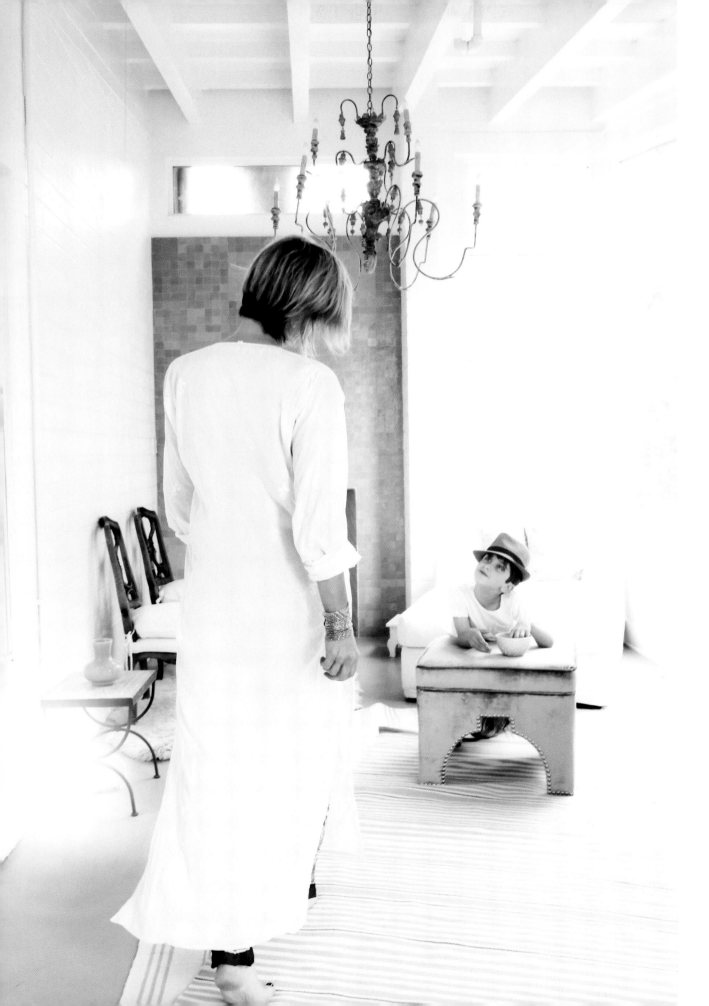

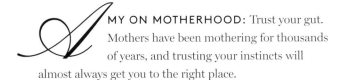

AMY ON MOTHERHOOD: Trust your gut. Mothers have been mothering for thousands of years, and trusting your instincts will almost always get you to the right place.

HARDEST PART: Watching my kids get hurt or into trouble. As a mom, your instinct is to comfort and protect them. When they get hurt on the soccer field my first instinct is "OK, we are done, let's go home, you don't need to play any more soccer today, or ever," but the truth is, they need to get back into the game if it's not serious. This is what helps to build resilient human beings.

BEST PART: Unconditional love. You can't imagine what it is until you have this human being that you put on this planet, whom you are completely responsible for. It made me redefine what love is.

LESSONS LEARNED: I read a funny quote that said, "I started to write a book on parenthood, and I ended up with a book of cocktail recipes." I am not saying that one should turn to the bottle for solace, but it's important to remember to still have fun and let go as mom.

HOME STYLE: *Whitewashed Beachy Meets Industrial*

PHILOSOPHY: Everything can be thrown in the wash or replaced. No one thing is more important than the people in my house.

Inspiration

The inspiration was "California modern meets New York loft." The whole renovation was risky. It's the kind of home where your reaction is that you have never seen anything quite like it—that kind of place could either be amazing or go terribly wrong. I designed the home to incorporate beautiful light all year long, with indoor/outdoor spaces to capture the true California lifestyle.

SECRETS OF DISGUISE: Designating a space for kids' toys that is easily accessible but not in view, and creating reward systems for cleaning up. I also incorporated lots of beautiful baskets and old trunks into the décor, as well as lots of shelves in their rooms.

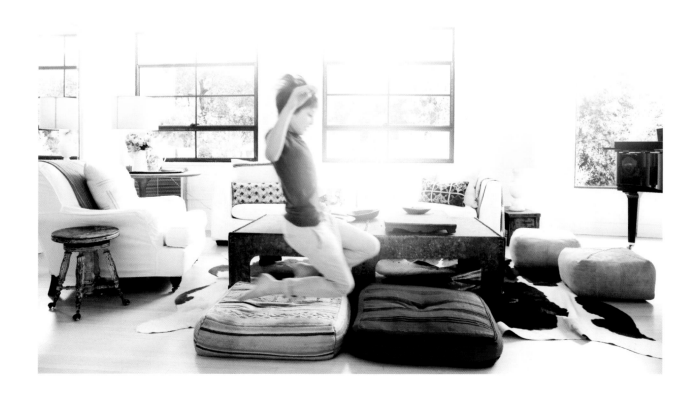

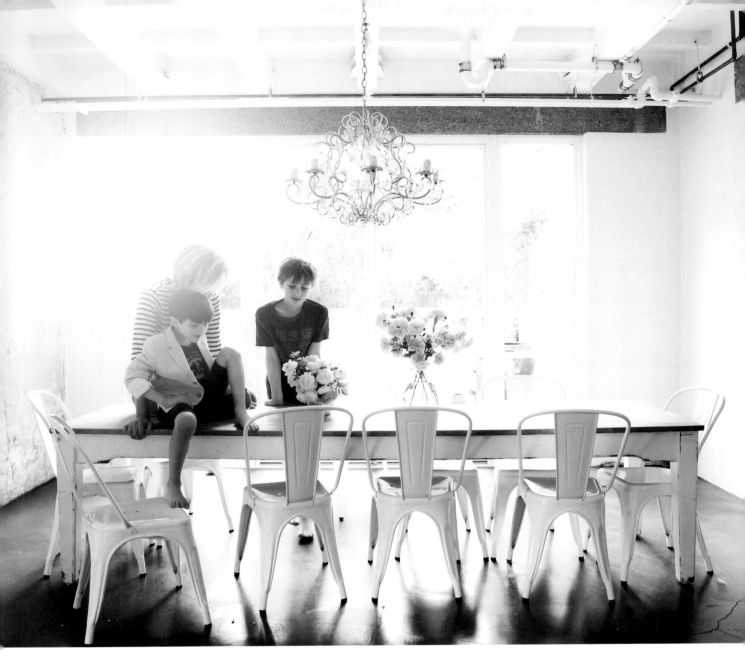

Save & Splurge

Save: Furniture, and lots of flea-market finds, like old farm tables.

Splurge: Lighting fixtures, surfaces, doors, and windows—because they are permanent.

DECORATING MANTRA: I never look for anything specific. I let the pieces speak to me.

MY HOME IS . . . Industrial, eclectic, a sanctuary . . . and always filled with friends and guests—it's beautifully chaotic most of the time. "Everyone is welcome" is our motto.

Resources

★ Greg Lauren painting
★ Dosa poof cushions
★ White couch from Buttercup, Culver City
★ Shabby Chic white roll arm chair
★ White table lamps from The Mart collective
★ Michel Ottin wood chairs
★ Dash & Albert striped layered rugs
★ Badia side table
★ One King's Lane studded ottoman
★ Shabby Chic chandelier
★ Pottery Barn dining chairs

Calgary AVANSINO

BRITISH *VOGUE* CONTRIBUTING EDITOR & HEALTH EXPERT

Daughters Ava Harlow and Margot Rae,
photographed at seven and three years old, respectively
London, England

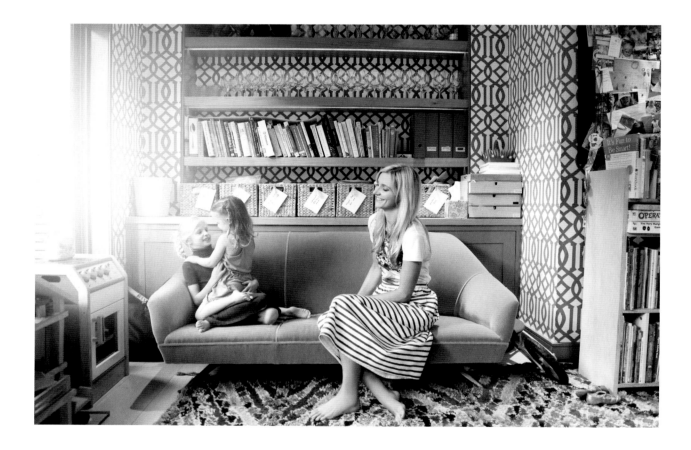

With her perfectly highlighted blond hair, mile-long legs, and to-die-for wardrobe, Calgary Avansino looks like the definition of effortless chic. But after spending five minutes with her, what becomes more striking than her seeming perfection is her humorous and endearingly sweet approach to motherhood. On the afternoon of our shoot, Avansino was getting ready for a Vogue event that evening, while still cooking her daughters a deliciously healthy dinner and letting them pick out her outfit for the night (they decided on a classic Michael Kors striped dress). At the core, she's a devoted mom determined to show her girls that hard work pays off.

CALGARY ON MOTHERHOOD: Being a mother makes you better at everything in your life: You're better at prioritizing; you're wiser, more self-confident; multitasking becomes second nature; and a crying baby on an airplane will never bother you again.

HARDEST PART: Learning how to control my temper and constructively navigate the inevitable turbulence (big and small) that arises.

BEST PART: Truly appreciating my own mother for the first time and all she did for me.

FAVORITE PART OF THE DAY: Right when I get home from work, they run to greet me with open arms, followed by a bath all together.

HOME STYLE: *Mid-Century Glamour*

PHILOSOPHY: Happiness must be at the core of the design—life is too short for beige.

Inspiration

My husband has a slight mid-century furniture addiction, which inspired the overall look of our home.

SECRETS OF DISGUISE: We have nearly as many baskets as we do toys. Throw everything in, and close the top.

HOMEMADE TOUCHES: I frame my children's art obsessively. I'm constantly on the hunt for vintage frames (I'm all about oval ones at the moment).

Save & Splurge

I'll buy an expensive piece of furniture and then follow it up by getting an old chair at a flea market for nothing and re-covering it. I have throw pillows in my house from IKEA that I love, next to elaborately embroidered cushions from Turkey. It's all about curating the mix.

Design Surprises

I upholstered our playroom couch in the most decadent orange silk velvet—I just couldn't resist, I loved the fabric so much. Even after countless spills and marker encounters it still looks striking and brings so much cheerfulness to the room. And we covered one entire wall of our sitting room in wood paneling—we weren't at all sure it was going to work aesthetically, but we loved it from the moment it was finished.

MY HOME IS . . . Vibrant, inviting, layered.

Resources

- ★ Kelly Wearstler Imperial Trellis wallpaper
- ★ Anthropologie rug

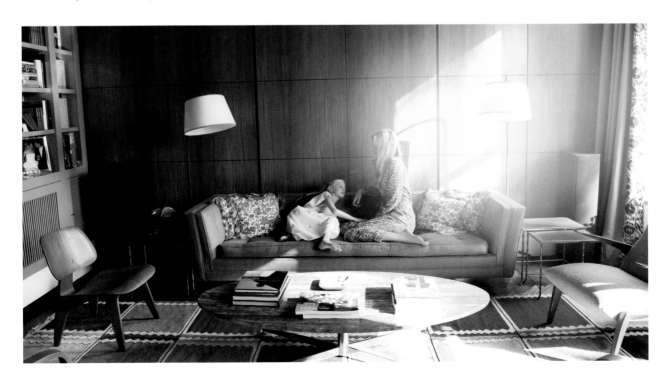

Jemma KIDD

BEAUTY EXPERT

Twins Arthur and Mae,
photographed at three years old
Reading, England

Jemma Kidd has been in the spotlight since the young age of sixteen. First, she began modeling (along with her sister, Jodie) before going on to win acclaim as an equestrian. Then, after much hard work and research, she launched her own makeup line, Jemma Kidd Beauty School. The cult-favorite brand became an international success. Now, as the mom of twins and the wife of Arthur, Earl of Mornington, Kidd (officially known as a countess) is more likely to be found on the grounds of her English country estate picking vegetables from her own garden in a pair of wellies than teetering around London in heels. She refers to herself as a country girl at heart, but her home reveals otherwise. While there are many classic country touches, like the roaring fireplaces and oversize furniture, the overall design goes way beyond traditional. In the end, Kidd accomplished what she set out to create: a "homey, comfortable, chic" house in which to raise her children.

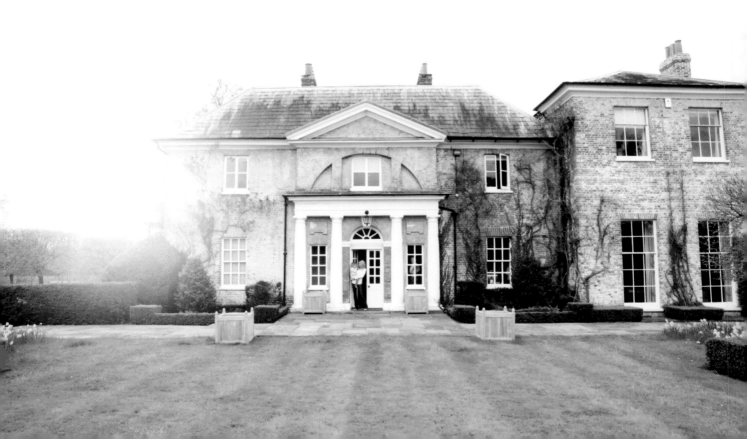

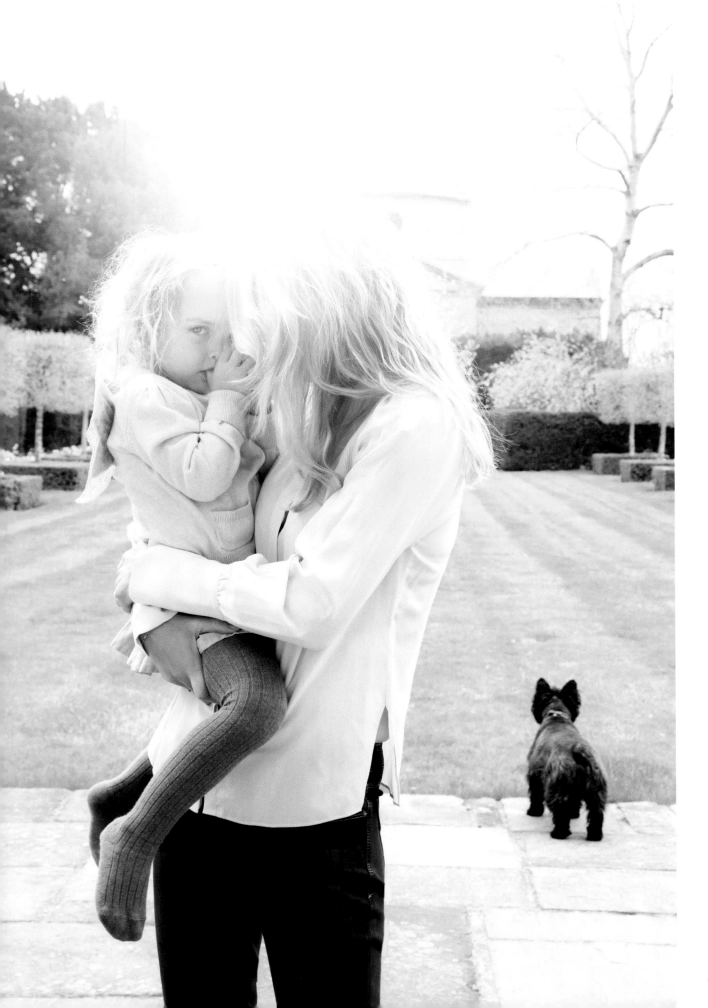

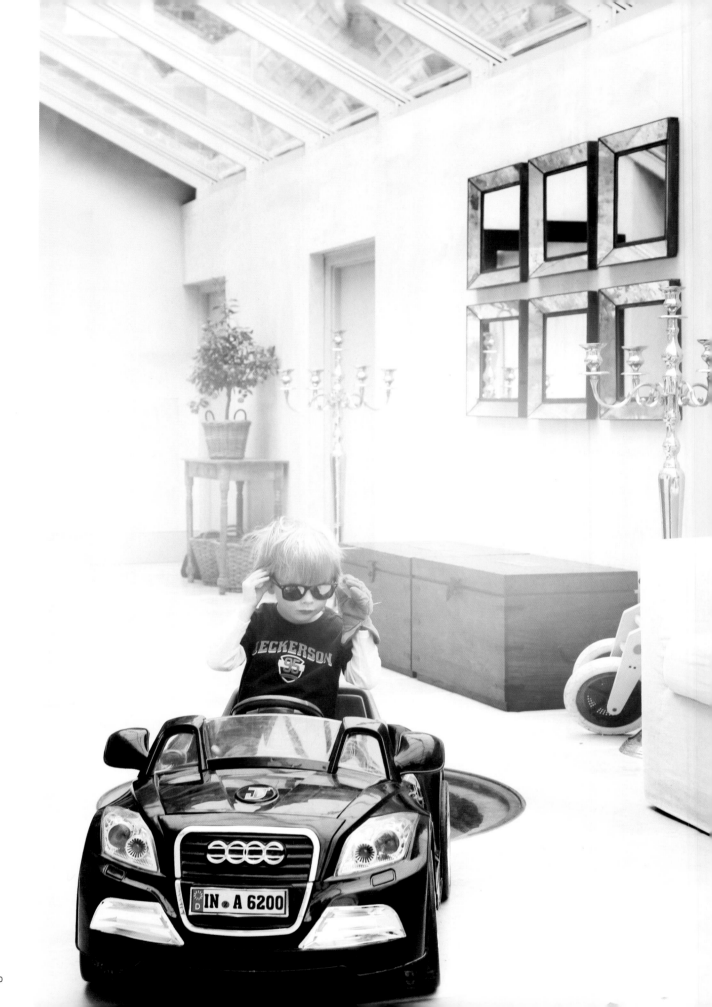

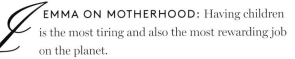

JEMMA ON MOTHERHOOD: Having children is the most tiring and also the most rewarding job on the planet.

HARDEST PART: Organizing: running the children's world, your world, your home, your work and also being a wife and happy hostess—plus, you want to look good on top of that!

BEST ADVICE: It's OK to ask for help—it doesn't mean you're a bad mother. I got a sleep trainer in to help me when lack of sleep was sending me over the edge.

FAVORITE PART OF THE DAY: Breakfast—we are all excited about the day ahead.

HOME STYLE: *Modern English Country*

PHILOSOPHY: It had to feel lived in and loved, so we filled it with oversize furniture, extremely comfortable soft furnishings, soft colors, thick curtains, and huge baths. I worked with Penny Morrison, who loves fabrics from India but can work them into a classic country house without it looking too themed.

Inspiration

I am a country girl at heart and love the whole look and feel of the country style. My husband's family had some wonderful bits of furniture and prints in the attic from his ancestral home, which we were able to incorporate into our home—each piece has such a unique style and history.

SECRETS OF DISGUISE: I like to have lots of storage: cupboards and storage boxes. And I have big wooden trunks, with big brass plaques with my children's names on them, which we put all their toys in. I am also really good at giving toys away to my friends and family—I find less is more. I've fallen in love with this divine company called the Great Little Trading Co. (www.gltc.co.uk)—it has the most wonderful solutions for storing your kids' toys, from table-top storage to toy-box storage. I love the pull-along book carts and the double stacking storage trunks. They have pieces you actually like to look at, which is pretty rare.

Design Surprises

We found a few interesting things while we were renovating, like a well in the courtyard (shown opposite). It's now covered with glass and lit, so it looks like a fun feature.

MY HOME IS . . . Homey, comfortable, chic.

Resources

* ★ Crate & Barrel mirrors
* ★ John Lewis wood trunks
* ★ Vintage wood table
* ★ OKA woven baskets

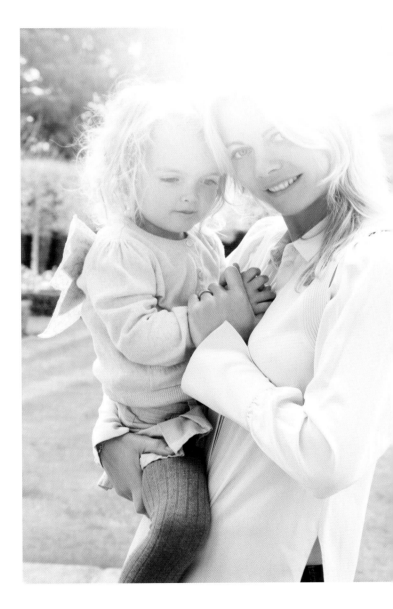

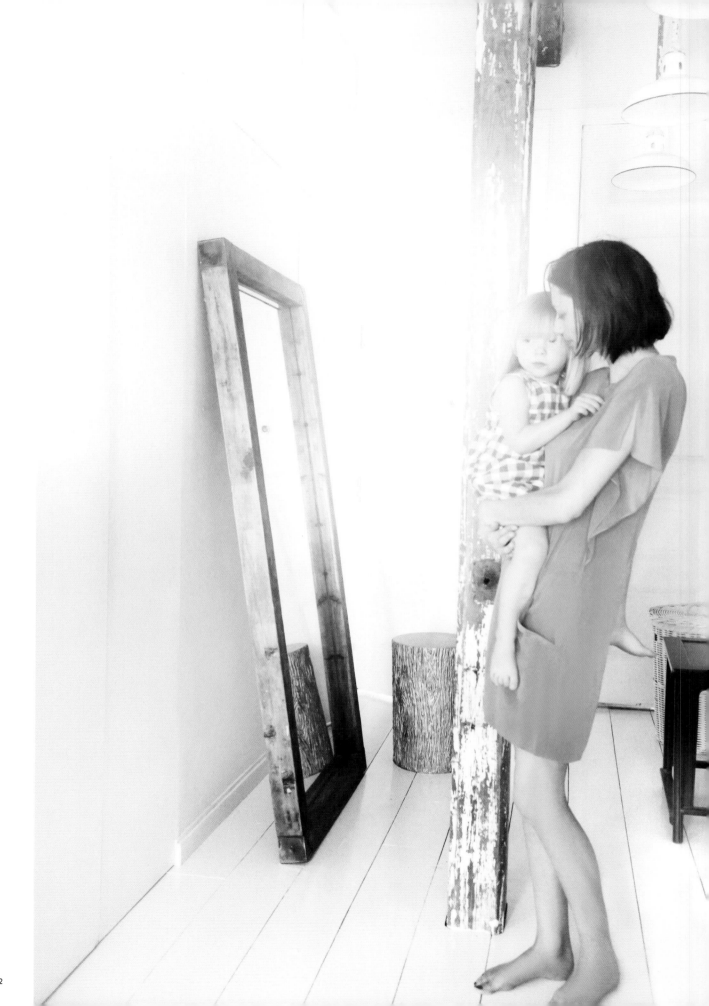

Kathryn NEALE

STYLIST

Son Eddie and daughter Frankie,
photographed at four and three years old, respectively
Brooklyn, New York

Vogue contributing editor Kathryn Neale is just as comfortable styling fashion shows for brands like Rebecca Minkoff and Peter Som as she is knee-deep in dirt in her beloved Brooklyn garden. When the New Zealand native first laid eyes on her current home, it was actually the slice of grass out back that sold her on the place. Since moving in, Neale has created a country-like oasis right in the heart of New York City—complete with wide-plank floors, exposed rustic beams, and a now-lush garden bursting with everything from roses to kale. Her two young children, brimming with polite charm (Neale takes manners very seriously), love to help their mom in the garden and even have their own veggies to tend to. And that's exactly how she likes it.

KATHRYN ON MOTHERHOOD: Reject the guilt. Enjoy what you are able to give as a wife and mother, and don't beat yourself up about the stuff you never actually get to (like the laundry).

FAVORITE PART: Being the most important person to somebody you adore, and being able to watch them develop with such intimacy.

MAMA TIP: I wish I was better at keeping their socks as pairs, so I recently started buying only black socks. This has been very effective.

FAVORITE PART OF THE DAY: Waking up: The kids come into our bed first thing and snuggle, then they get bored and start opening our eyelids or sticking fingers up our noses. It sounds annoying, but it's the best alarm clock.

HOME STYLE: *Rustic Country Charm*

Inspiration

I wanted the kitchen to be the heart of the home, and the focus to be on the garden.

THE STARTING POINT: The salvaged beams our architect found at a wreck yard.

BIGGEST CHALLENGE: I am always trying to keep our house empty, and now there are two more opponents in my battle. I'm losing the battle against stuff, and I'm kind of OK with it. I tend to buy them books as opposed to toys, and chuck out the noisy toys whenever they aren't looking.

MOST PERSONAL: I love my husband's old couch—it's been with him longer than I have (at least fifteen years). He really wants to get it reupholstered, but I love its faded glory.

IN THE GARDEN: My kids love to help me in the garden, and each have their own veggies that they're growing. All you have to do with toddlers is invite them to work with you and keep them interested.

MY HOME IS . . . Cool, lush, and full of good food aromas.

Resources

* West Elm tree trunk stool
* Mirror from the Brooklyn Flea

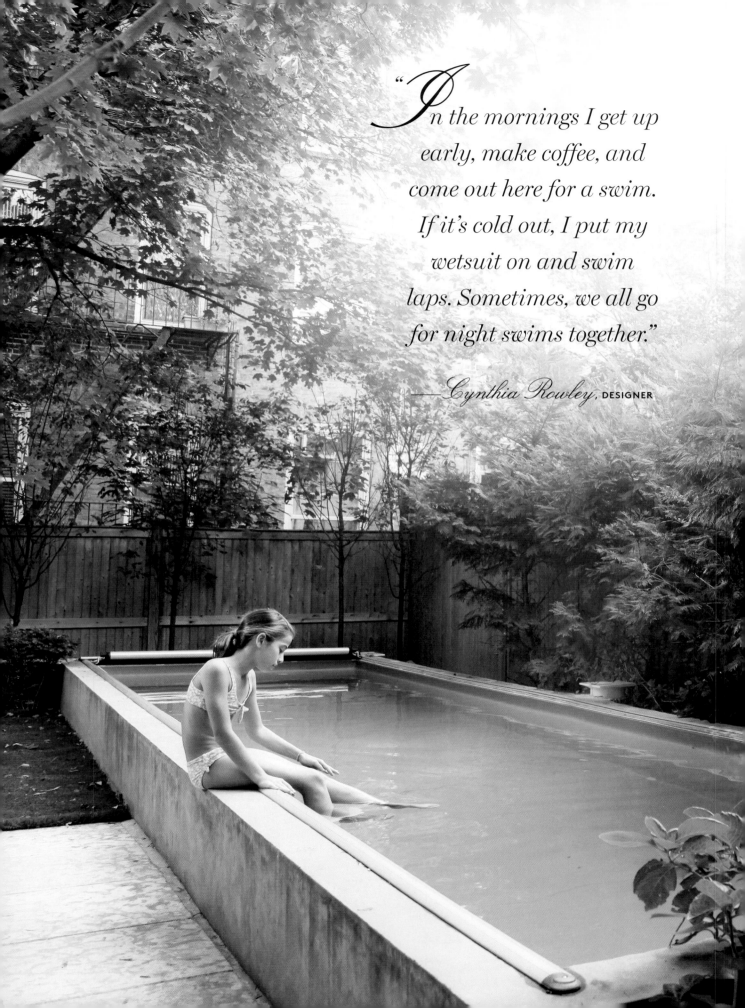

"*In the mornings I get up early, make coffee, and come out here for a swim. If it's cold out, I put my wetsuit on and swim laps. Sometimes, we all go for night swims together.*"

—Cynthia Rowley, DESIGNER

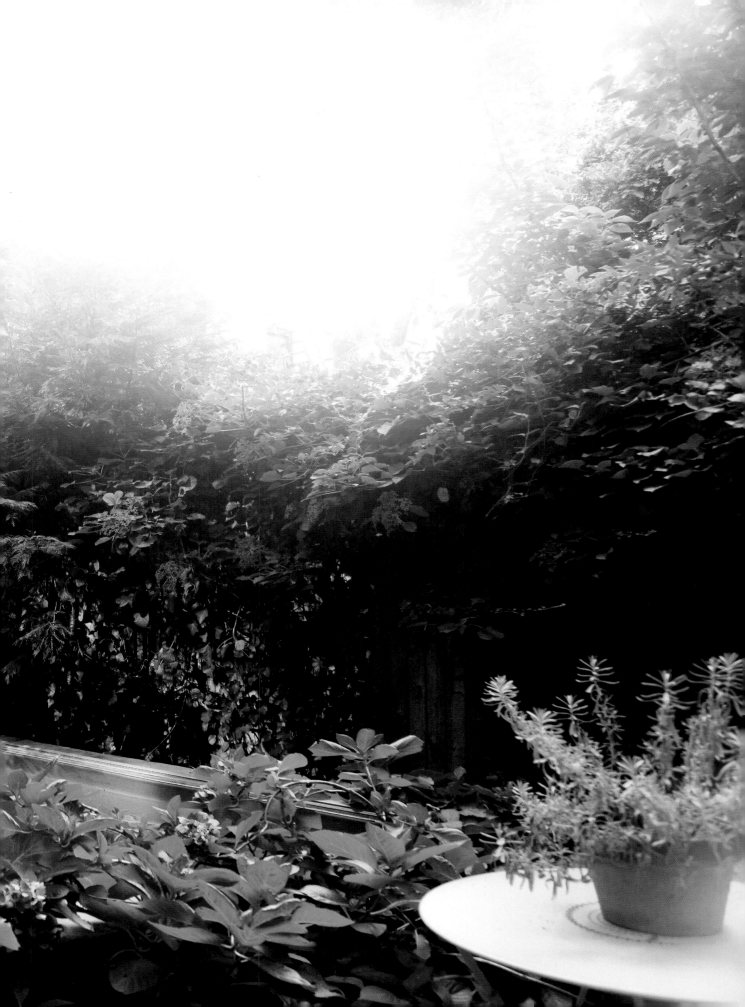

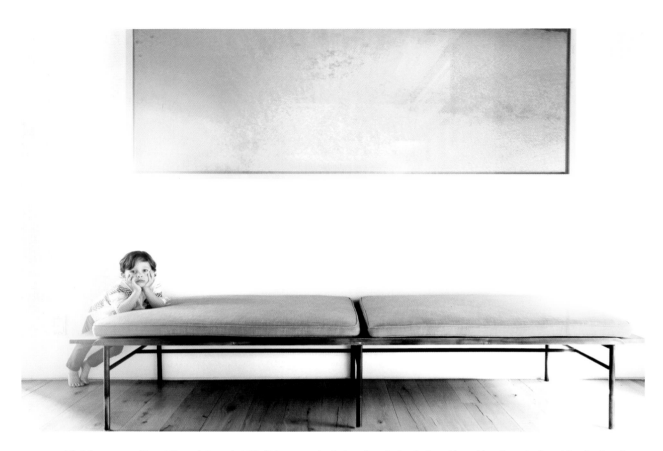

ABOVE: A bright corner of Jenni Kayne's Beverly Hills living room includes a bench she designed herself, and a print by Richard Misrach.
BELOW: Kayne's custom built-in bench provides comfy, informal seating in her open kitchen.

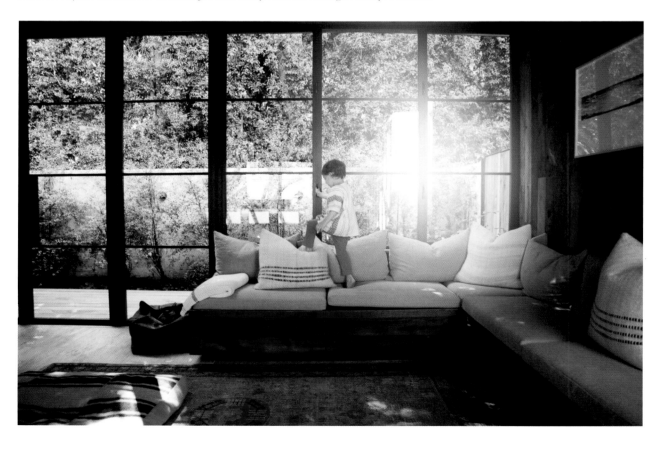

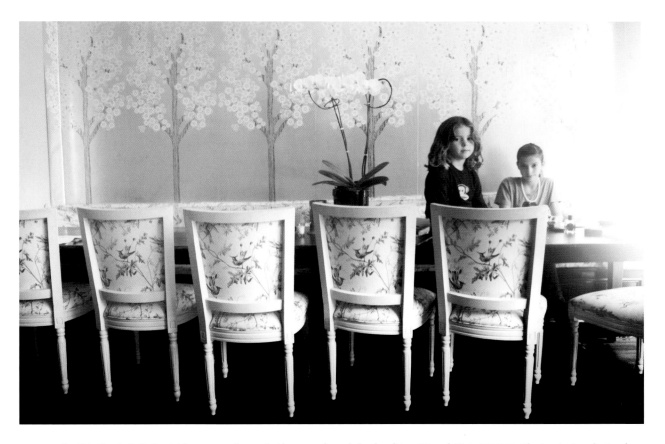

ABOVE: Cynthia Rowley's dining table serves as the perfect homework nook for daughters Kit and Gigi. BELOW: The inspiration for jewelry designer Lynn Ban's Manhattan apartment was a modern hotel suite, and the starting point was this floor-to-ceiling built-in bookshelf.

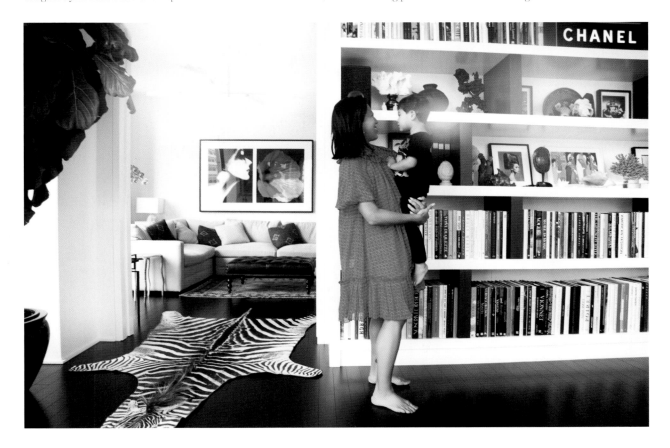

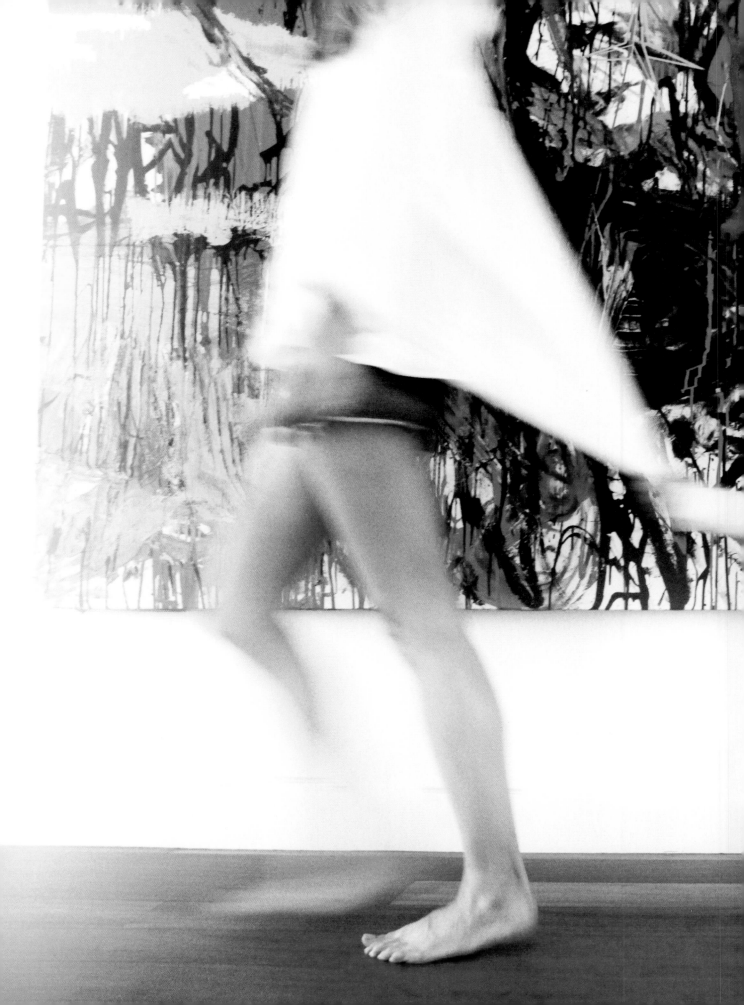

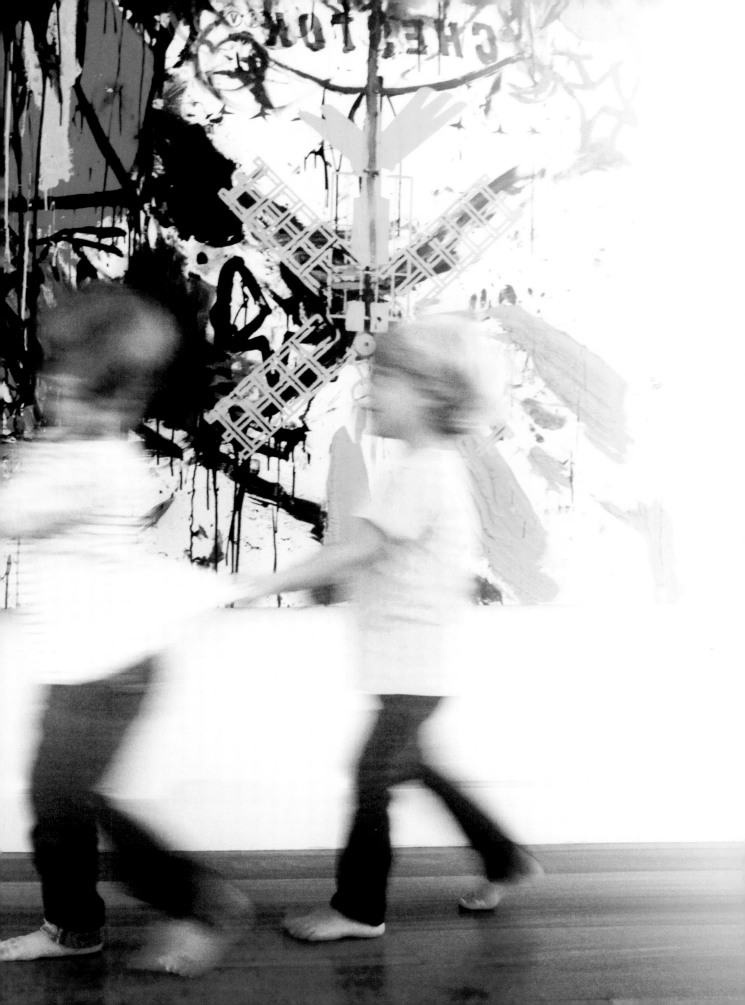

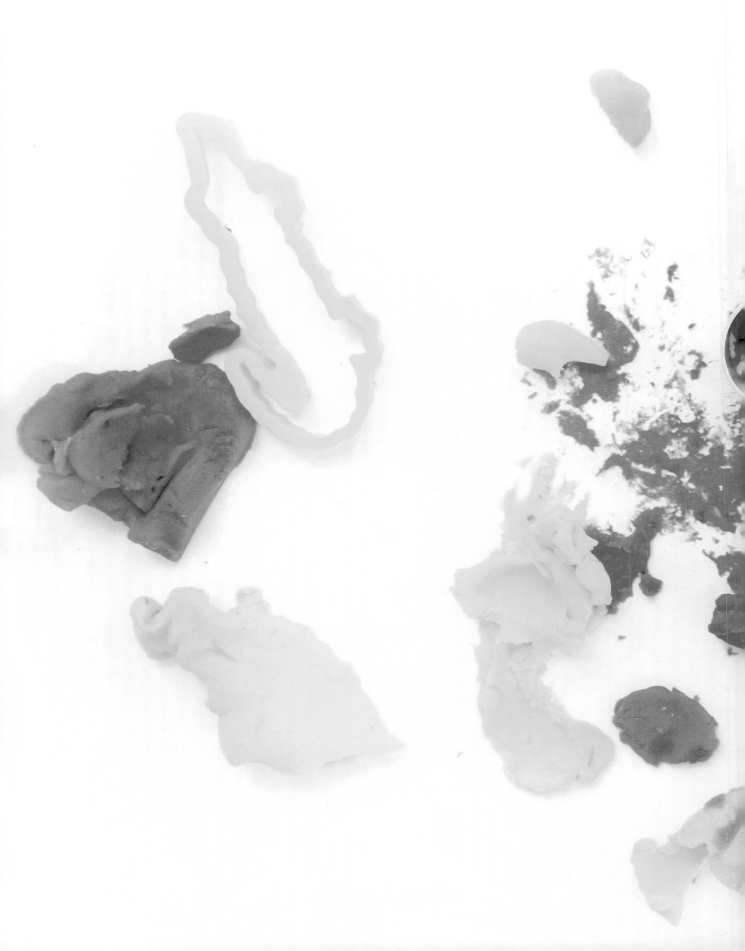

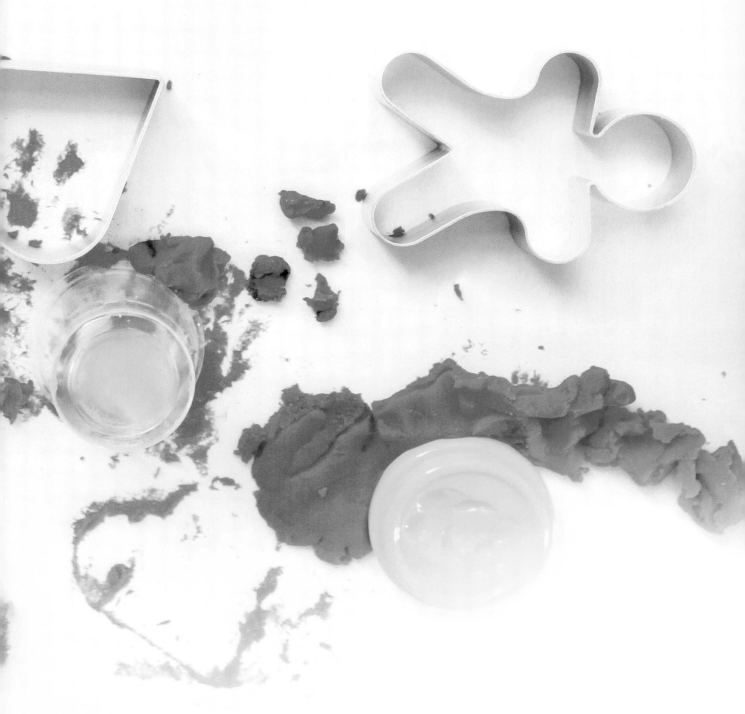

CHAPTER FIVE

The Essentials

ZOË BUCKMAN, *photographer* · SIMONE HAROUCHE, *stylist & designer*

RACHELLE HRUSKA, *cofounder of Guest of a Guest* · MARYAM NASSIR ZADEH, *boutique owner & designer*

AND MORE. . .

While many soon-to-be moms, myself included, start out with the lofty notion of curating a minimal-chic collection of baby "stuff," as reality (and your child's needs) sets in, the practicality of motherhood often wins out. That said, it is entirely possible to zero in on what's important and weed out the excess (baby wipes warmer, anyone?). When it came time to stock up on basics for my baby, I took this advice from Christina Hutson to heart: "Buy the necessities, and wait and see what you and your baby love and need—you will never know until the moment arrives." Deciding to keep things simple and only buying the bare minimum to start with was a win-win situation—not only was my small apartment less cluttered, I also felt lighter and more focused going into new motherhood. My list of must-haves was culled from The Glow archives and countless e-mails with the in-the-know moms who have appeared on the site. The curated list they helped me create—filled with everything from the perfect baby carrier to the softest stuffed animals—saved me time, space, and money. In this chapter, we share with you some of our essentials, including the beloved books, activities, and toys that will keep your child stimulated and entertained, starting with the newborn phase and beyond.

All it takes is one look at Pinterest to get completely inspired, and then quickly over-whelmed, by the plethora of baby and kids' gear out there—from eco-friendly wooden toys to life-changing swaddle blankets. Weeding through the good, the bad, and the totally unneces-sary can feel like a part-time job. Rachelle Hruska, for one, is partial to wooden toys. As the Guest of a Guest cofounder explains, "I like the idea that they may someday be passed down to my son's kids. Hopefully they'll hold up over time, like some of my old toys that my parents have given back to me."

Photographer Zoë Buckman agrees: "I really like crocheted or wooden toys for my daugh-ter. They're old-fashioned, pretty, and have been working for years, so why change it up and get flashy plastic toys?"

Boutique owner Maryam Nassir Zadeh learned early on that banning certain toys from her daughter was a losing battle. "I want to make ugly toys off-limits, but I don't have the heart to do that," she says. And on the upside, "Most of it is temporary, and we won't keep them long term."

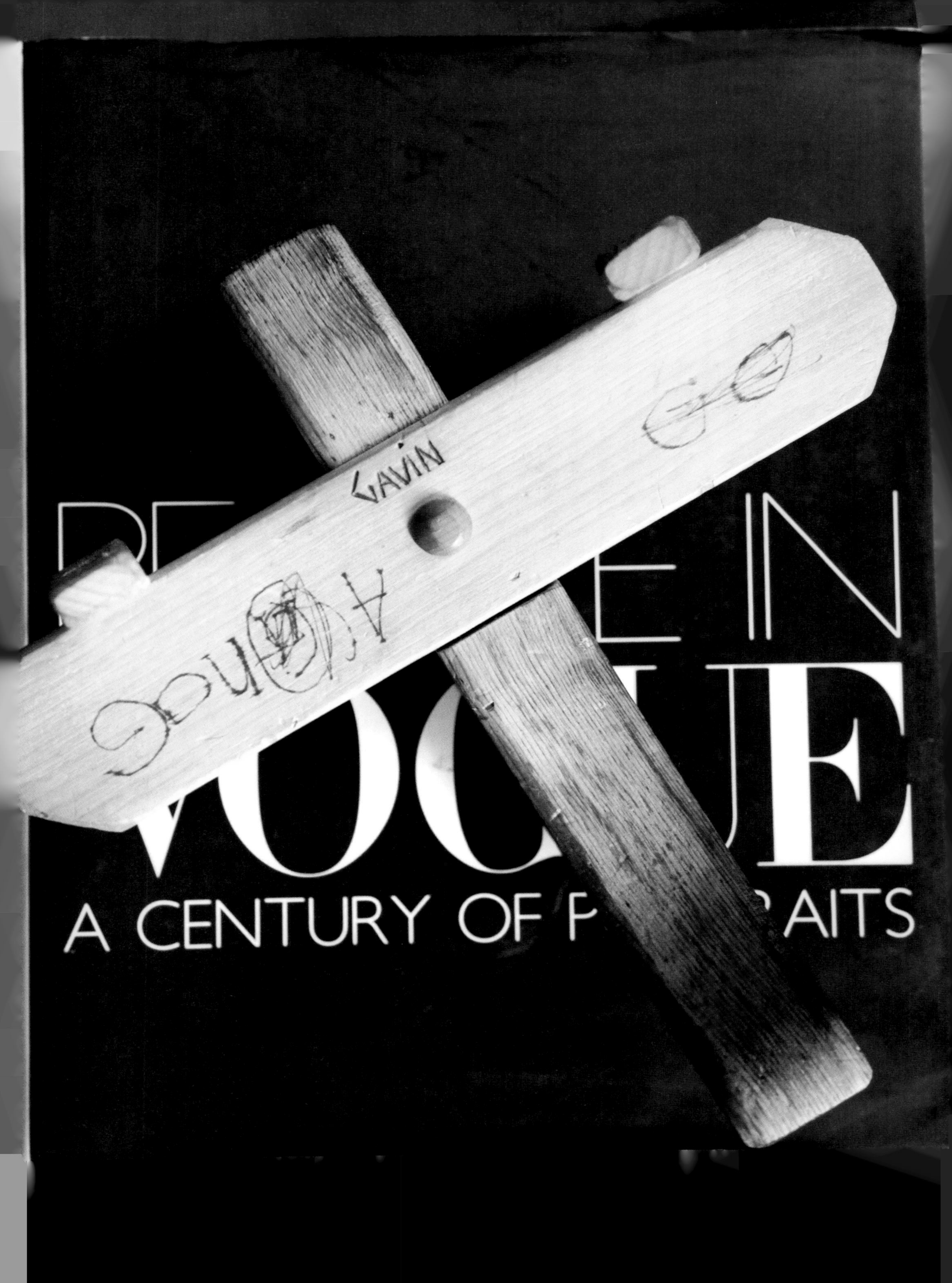
GAVIN
IN
A CENTURY OF

Zoë BUCKMAN

Daughter Cleo, photographed at seven months old
New York, New York

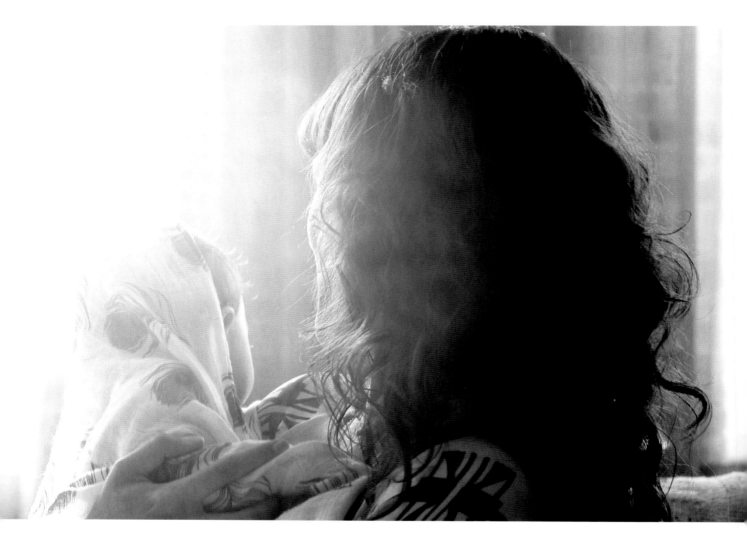

The story of photographer Zoë Buckman reads like a modern-day fairy tale, only more superhero than Cinderella: After only a few years in New York, she snagged her first solo show at Milk Studios, then married her long-time love, the actor and director David Schwimmer, followed by the birth of their first child, and then on to the gut renovation of a brownstone. A native of East London, Buckman splits her time between shooting features for *Marie Claire* and *GQ* and doting on her daughter, Cleo. For Buckman, motherhood has been all about balance—tea and biscuits in the morning and sweet Manhattans after Cleo's gone to bed.

ZOË ON MOTHERHOOD: I thought that I was loving with all of my heart before, but now that I have a child I've discovered a whole new depth of love (for my kid, my husband, my parents).

HARDEST PART: You experience fear and sorrow in greater depth. As morbid as it sounds, the hardest thing about being a mum is the sudden awareness of my and my child's mortality.

BEST ADVICE: As she left our house after I'd given birth, my midwife told me to trust my instincts—it's proved invaluable.

Playtime

CLEO'S FIRST TOY: When I was pregnant, I slept with these two stuffed animal bunnies with the hope that they would take on my scent and be a comfort to her when she was first born (they were also nice cushions for my big belly). Now she loves them and can't sleep without them.

ZOË'S FAVORITE TOYS: For my own sanity and selfishness, I've tried to avoid plastic toys, especially those that make obnoxious noises (which, of course, she loves). So I've had to give in to one or two. I'm quite adamant about not giving her toys that perpetuate impossible standards of beauty or that reinforce a male sexual ideal, like Barbie. I'm not thrilled with the idea of her playing with toys that reinforce female stereotypes either, like cleaning or cooking, though I realize parents can take this too far. I'm happy for her to pretend to make tea and bake, as long as it's countered with creative play. It also helps that her dad will play with all of these things with her, too, so that she won't associate certain activities as being just for women.

BOOKS: I love reading her *Each Peach Pear Plum*, *Time for Bed*, and *Planting a Rainbow*, which is about planting flowers and naming the colors. As a child, I loved *The Tiger Who Came to Tea*, *Happy Birthday, Moon*, *Winnie the Pooh*, *Burglar Bill*, and *In the Night Kitchen*. I'm just starting to read these to her.

ACTIVITIES: I love pavement crayons because we can go outside and do things like draw hopscotch on the ground, which helps her repeat her numbers. I love doing anything artistic with her—coloring, painting, making things out of clay. Hide-and-seek with her has me in hysterics, too.

Zoë's Essentials

* A hands-free device for your mobile phone
* A cross-body bag or backpack
* A camera that can easily switch to video
* Some kind of gift to yourself every day—a bath, cup of tea, magazine, nap—something that's just for you

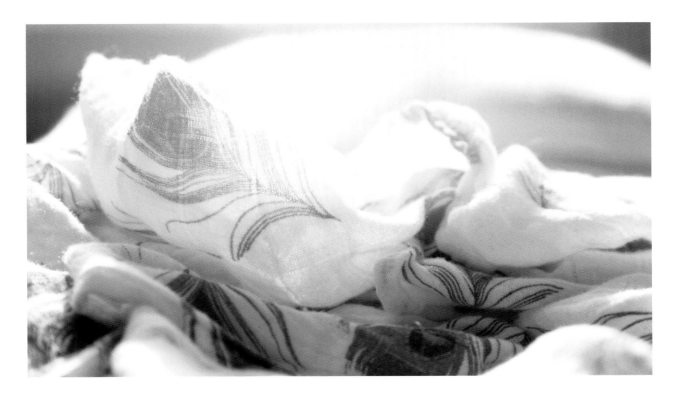

Simone HAROUCHE

STYLIST & DESIGNER

———————

Son Dashiel,
photographed at seven months old
Los Angeles, California

With her pale blond hair and lightly bronzed skin, Simone Harouche embodies classic California style, right down to her enviable collection of perfectly frayed denim shorts. Her busy life as a stylist (to stars like Christina Aguilera and Miley Cyrus) and designer of her own boho-chic handbag collection, Simone Camille, has slowed down only slightly since her son, Dashiel, entered the world. To counterbalance the hectic nature of her not-so-nine-to-five job, Harouche has created an eclectic home for her family that is at once serene and vibrant. For her son's nursery, she poured her heart and soul into the highly personal design, filling the space with pieces picked up on her world travels. A self-proclaimed neat freak, she admits that she runs a tight ship when it comes to sleep time and organization. Her goal: "To keep our house from looking like one giant playroom." So far, mission accomplished.

SIMONE ON MOTHERHOOD: I try not to judge myself or be too hard on myself for the choices I make as a mom. I make mistakes a lot, but I live and learn from them. I am constantly striving to be a better woman and mother and consider myself a work in progress.

BIGGEST SURPRISE: How little time there is in a day to get everything done. And how hard it is (in the beginning) to get yourself together and out of the house before two p.m.

HARDEST PART: Learning how to be really present with my son. I try to be conscious about how much I am on my iPhone or computer around him, but have become so accustomed to always being attached to some form of communication. Now that I'm a mom, it's nice to sometimes disconnect and be in the moment with Dashiel. I don't want to miss his childhood because I was too busy to look up from my phone.

FAVORITE PART OF THE DAY: In the morning, when the world is still quiet and we get to share these little moments together. We always start the day at seven a.m., so whether I walk into his room and find him sitting up in his crib or I have to wake him up, once he opens his eyes, he always greets me with the biggest smile. It fills my heart up to see him with that big happy smile.

GREATEST LESSON LEARNED: This too shall pass.

Playtime

DASHIEL'S FIRST TOY: While I was pregnant with Dash, I took a trip to Paris with my best friend. While we were there, we did some major baby shopping. The first toy I bought him was a stuffed toy musical guitar—it's covered in really cool printed fabrics, and when you pull the string, it plays "Twinkle, Twinkle, Little Star."

SIMONE'S FAVORITE TOYS: I really like the Lamaze soft development toys for him, and wooden musical toys. I try to avoid plastic toys, so I haven't bought any for him personally. But my parents and my husband's parents don't see the problem in them and buy him lots of plastic toys that talk to him and light up—they are insane, but Dash loves them. As he gets older, I am going to try my hardest to keep him away from toy weapons—I just don't get plastic guns.

Simone's Essentials

- ★ Calendula cream for skin irritations and diaper rash
- ★ Camomilla (homeopathic medicine) for teething and irritability
- ★ Cocyntal (homeopathic medicine) for colic and gas
- ★ Under the Nile layettes
- ★ Snap-N-Go (lightweight stroller for the infant car seat)
- ★ For sleep time: white noise, blackout shades, and Angel Dear lovies (they are a real lifesaver)
- ★ Custom-made Simone Camille diaper bag
- ★ Jellycat soft books

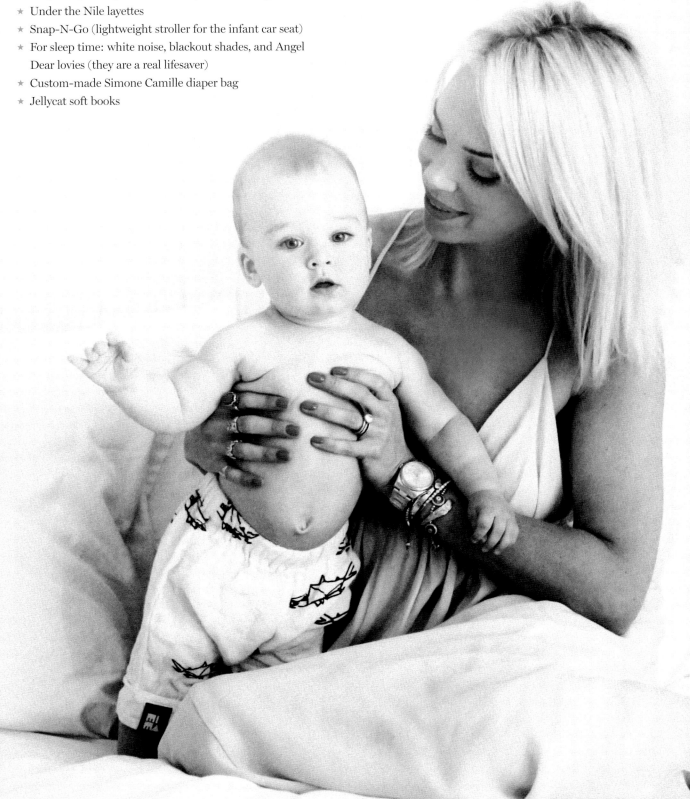

Rachelle HRUSKA

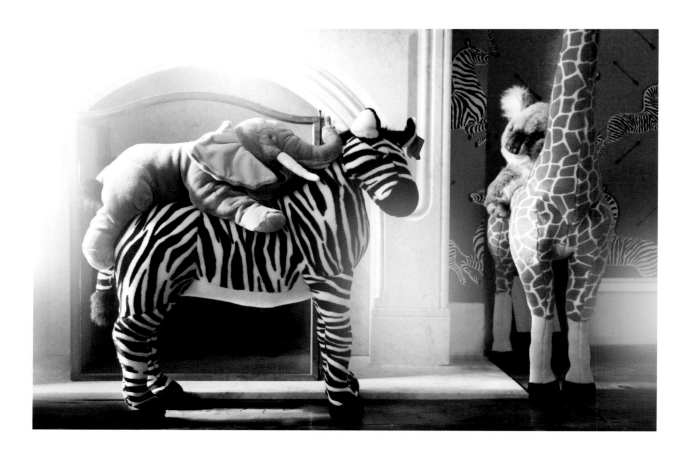

Since arriving in New York eight years ago, Rachelle Hruska has lived life in overdrive. The Internet entrepreneur and mom went from fresh-faced Midwesterner to mini mogul in just a few short years after cofounding social nightlife and event site Guest of a Guest (launched in 2008 with Cameron Winklevoss of Facebook fame). Life began to change even more drastically when Hruska was introduced to hotelier Sean McPherson (owner of The Bowery in Manhattan and the Crow's Nest in Montauk, among many others). Friendship turned into a whirl-wind romance, and marriage and baby soon followed. Hruska's priorities may have shifted, but she's far from slowing down—if anything, she's more focused and motivated than ever. As the first-time mom puts it, "Every day is a little more regimented, but it's beautiful—I'm having the most fun I've ever had in my whole life."

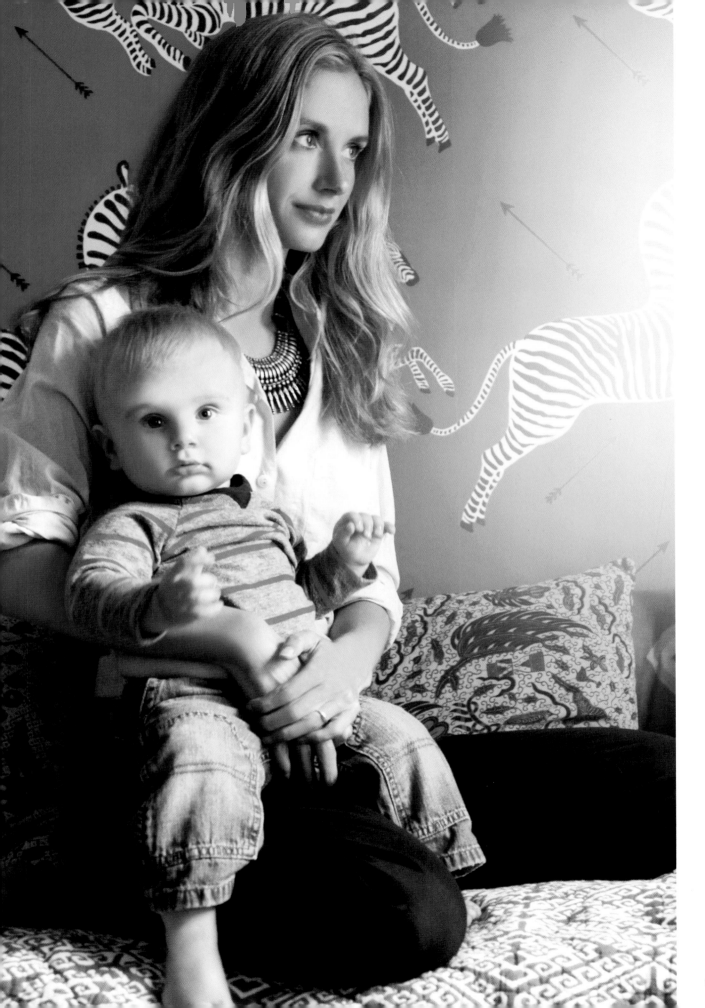

RACHELLE ON MOTHERHOOD: Every single day is an adventure. I have a very emotionally supportive husband, and that is everything. When you have someone who's saying, "You go and rock it," you feel like you can do anything. Our friend Bill Powers, Cynthia Rowley's husband, told us that the first six months of being a parent are like life support: They hang out and almost literally take all of you. I woke up the other day and said, "I can't believe Maxwell is eight months old—we made it this far."

HARDEST PART: The heaviness of it all. Life was much lighter when I didn't have to worry about another person so intimately.

BEST PART: The heaviness of it all. Life is so much better knowing that I get to have the most intimate of connections that humans are capable of having. That goes for my relationship with my husband as well as with my son. My husband and I have grown so much throughout this process—everything else seems so trivial in comparison.

Playtime

MAXWELL'S FAVORITE TOYS: His first favorite toys were the Jellycat soft books.

RACHELLE'S FAVORITE TOYS: I'm partial to wooden toys. I like the idea that they may someday be passed down to Maxwell's kids. Hopefully they'll hold up over time, like some of my old toys that my parents have given back to me. We soon found out that as a baby, he gravitated toward anything that lit up or made noise, and as much as we wanted to keep plastic off-limits, he ended up with his share of synthetic toys.

BOOKS: I love reading him my childhood favorites, like the Dr. Seuss books, because they are fun to read and remind me of being a child. His favorite right now is *Run, Dogs, Run!*

Rachelle's Essentials

* A Moses basket: We didn't use anything else for the first three months.
* A well-stocked iPhone: It helped me from getting bored while breast-feeding.
* Jellycat stuffed animals: So soft!
* Mustela bath products
* Any touch-and-feel book for baby
* Tata Harper face lotion: For me! It's expensive but feels so luxe, which is really important after delivering a baby.

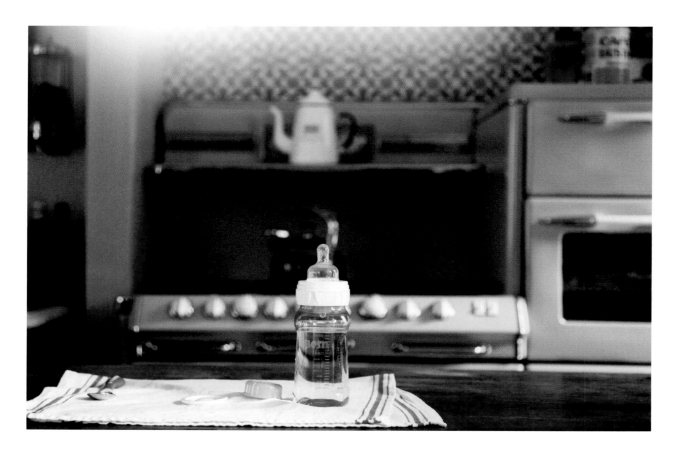

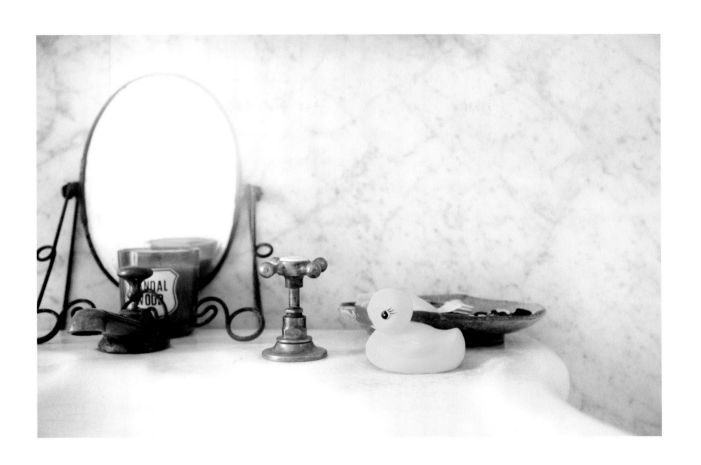

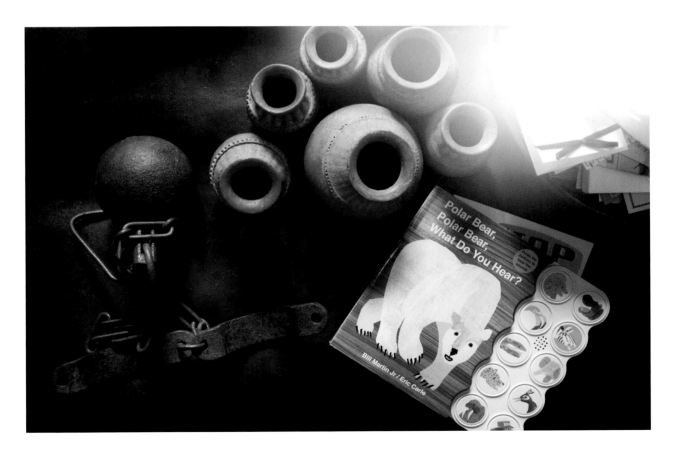

Maryam NASSIR ZADEH

BOUTIQUE OWNER & DESIGNER

Daughter Anaïs Vida,
photographed at two years old
New York, New York

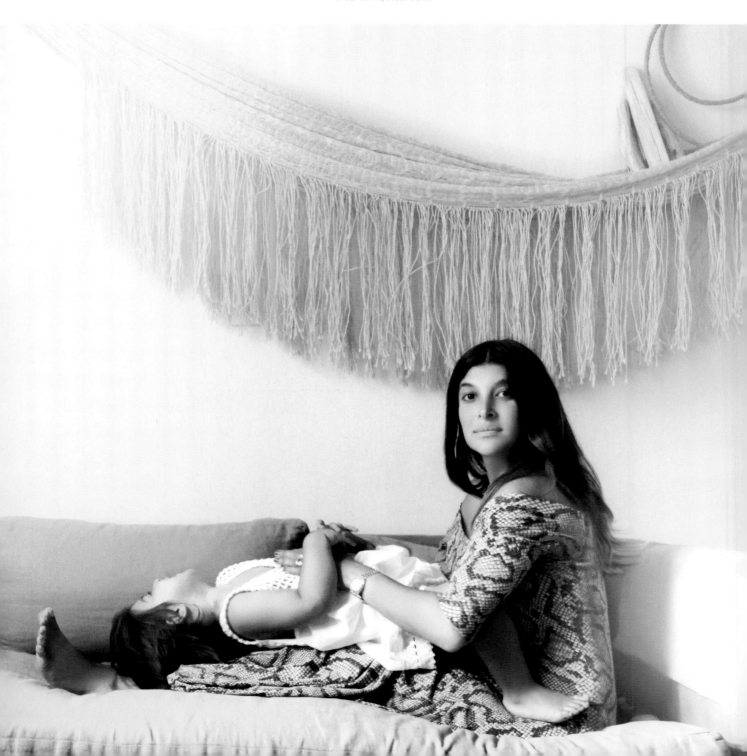

Known for her impeccably curated, globally inspired downtown boutique, Maryam Nassir Zadeh applies the same level of discernment to her personal and home décor style. Much like her store (a favorite of in-the-know women with an eye for the unexpected), the Iran-born beauty has filled her home with treasured finds from Mexico, India, and Montauk. But for this growing family, staying in one place too long is not in the cards. Before the birth of their second daughter, the close-knit clan traded in the busy streets of Manhattan for the palm trees and bougainvillea of Los Angeles (where Zadeh grew up). Considering their adventurous spirits and nomadic style, we have a feeling that wherever they hang their hats will instantly become home.

MARYAM ON MOTHERHOOD: I was once told by an astrologer that you and your child pick each other before they are born. It's incredible to think we are destined to live our lives together, and that my children will be my friends forever. It's the best feeling to experience building your own family—these are the most significant relationships you have in life.

HARDEST PART: As overwhelming as motherhood might be at times, everything falls into place and has its space to exist. The more you open your life to opportunities and experiences, the more life makes room for the abundance.

FAVORITE PART OF THE DAY: Anaïs stays up very late and sleeps with us in our bed, so we don't get tons of private time! Right before she's about to fall asleep, she puts her leg around my husband and her arm around my neck and gets really cozy and loving. It's always the best moment to feel the day is winding down with three of us all experiencing love together. She really feels connected to us, and nothing could give me more satisfaction.

Playtime

ANAÏS'S FIRST TOY: A stuffed bunny from Bonpoint.

MARYAM'S FAVORITE TOYS: I want to make ugly toys off-limits, but I don't have the heart to do that; I know they are temporary, and we won't keep them long term. She has

plastic dolls, Barbies, dinosaurs, and little doll-furniture pieces, which my mom bought for her. Even if there's a toy I'm not crazy about, I've noticed that it isn't a huge problem because she really rotates her toys and loves discovering new ones. She ends up playing with a variety of materials, and I find it hard to avoid plastic altogether. Everything I personally buy her is wooden or textile based, and at her Montessori school she is exposed to wooden and natural toys on a daily basis, so I'm not too concerned.

BOOKS: My favorite book to read to her is *Love You Forever*. Her favorite book is *My Friends*, by Taro Gomi.

Maryam's Essentials

* ★ Co-sleeper
* ★ Ergobaby carrier
* ★ Bugaboo Cameleon and Bugaboo Bee
* ★ Portable changing pad
* ★ Little stuffed animal
* ★ Tons of onesies
* ★ Dr. Brown's bottles
* ★ Mustela products

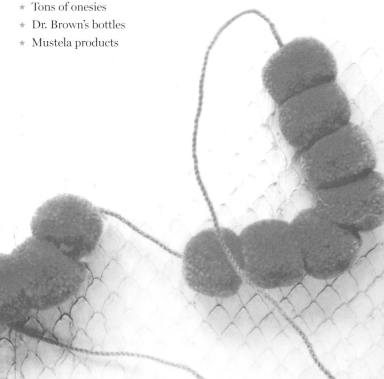

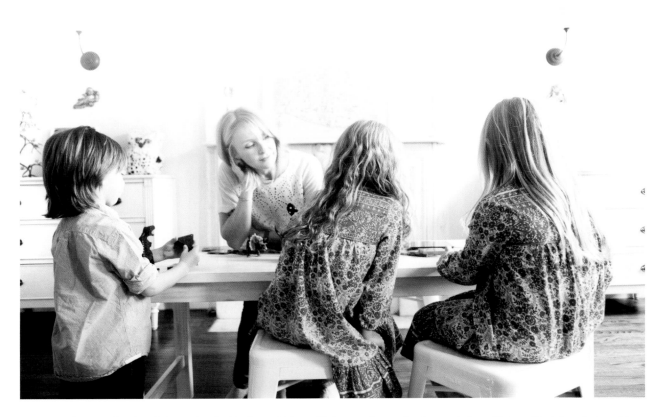

ABOVE: In her twin daughters' vintage-inspired bedroom, Rebecca Taylor spends countless hours playing with two of their favorite toys: Magna-Tiles and dinosaurs. BELOW: Jeanine Lobell's daughter Esme knits Rodarte-like throw blankets for her Manhattan bedroom.

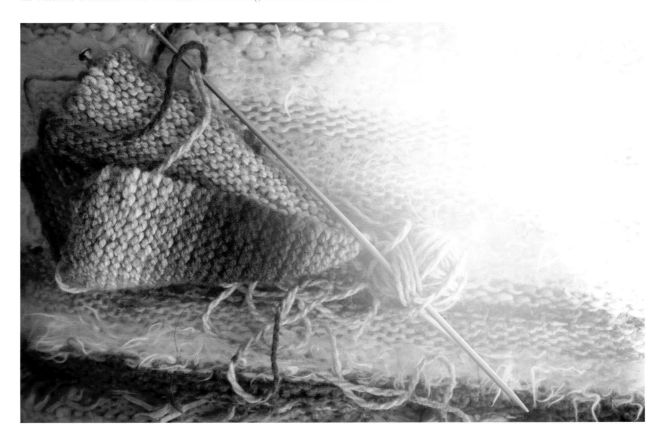

THE ESSENTIALS

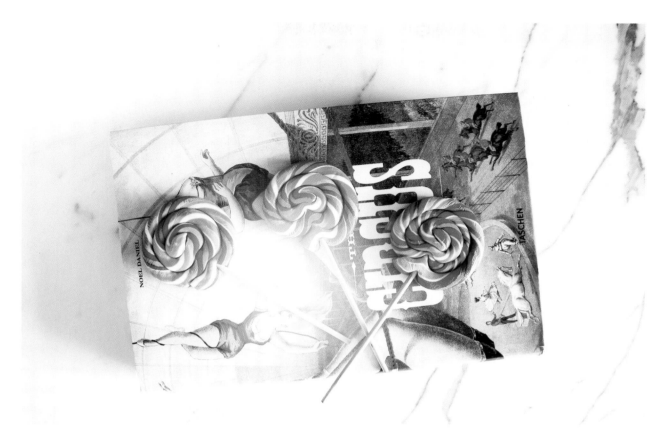

ABOVE: An unexpected mix of lollipops and art on Sara Blakely's living room bar—a crowd pleaser for both mom and her little one. BELOW: This bright Skip Hop play mat adds a bold pop of color, and endless entertainment, to Ana Lerario-Geller's mostly white living room.

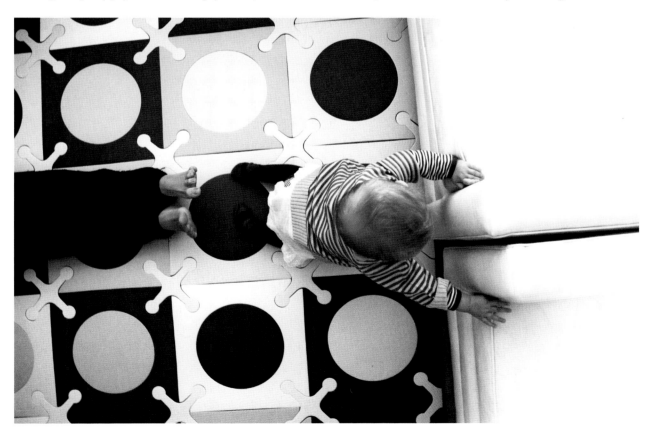

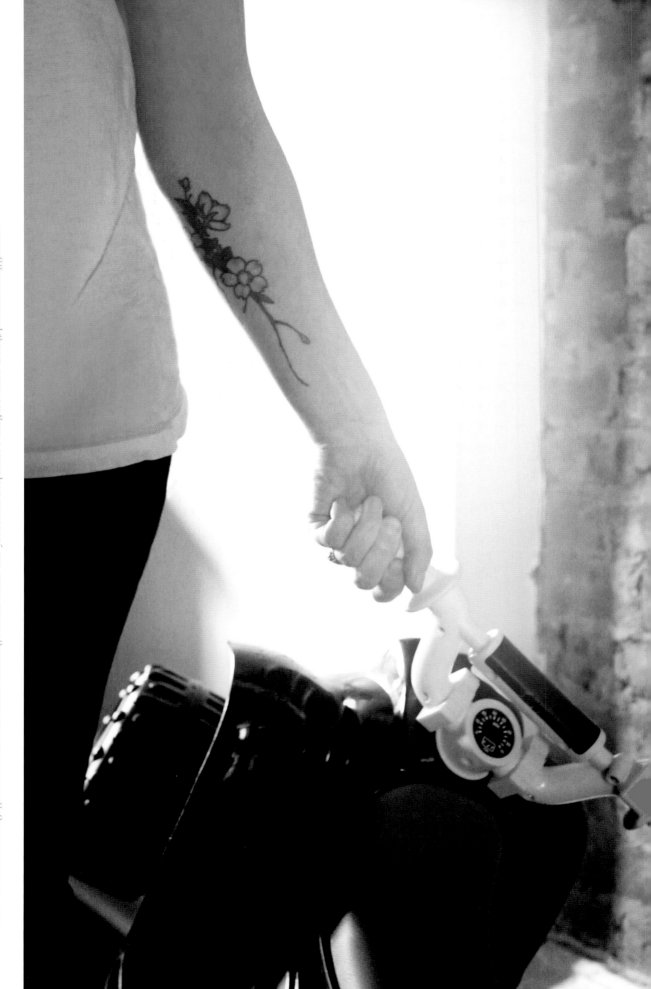

RIGHT: In-demand casting agent Anita Bitton has learned that being a mother means that "you become a superhero overnight. A multi-tasking, problem solving goddess."

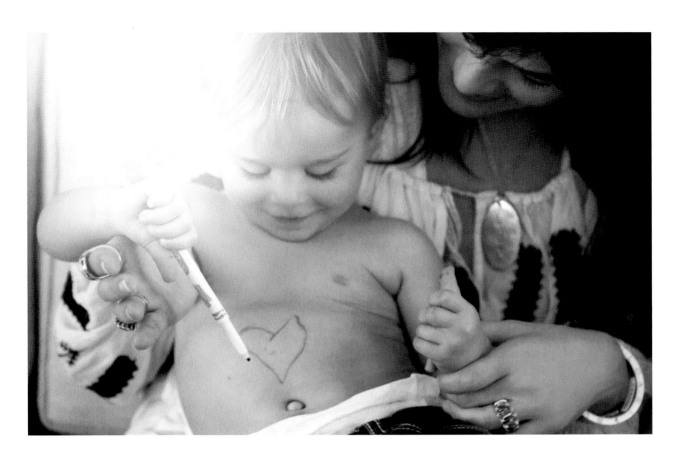

ABOVE: Selma Blair and son Arthur give each other temporary love "tattoos." BELOW: The photo booth in Busy Philipps's Los Angeles home provides endless entertainment for her daughter Birdie, and a fun collage wall displays all the photos they've taken with friends and family.

PHOTOS

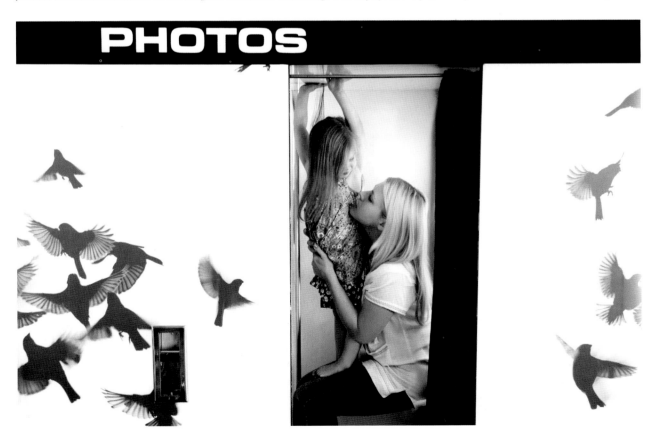

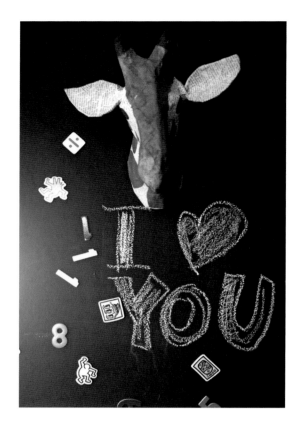

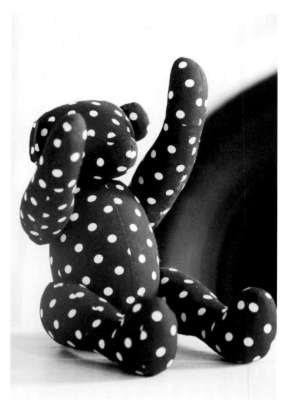

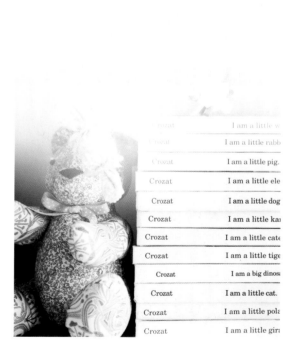

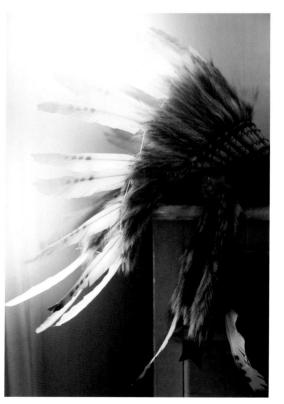

CLOCKWISE FROM TOP LEFT: A playful mix of stickers, animals, and a sweet message cover the chalkboard paint-covered wall in Christina Hutson's son's bedroom; Rebecca Taylor accessorizes her twin daughters' bedroom with a Comme des Garçons teddy bear; Caroline Deroche Pasquier's son Martin proudly displays this native American headdress in his Paris bedroom; a stack of Francois Crozat books in Calgary Avansino's London home.

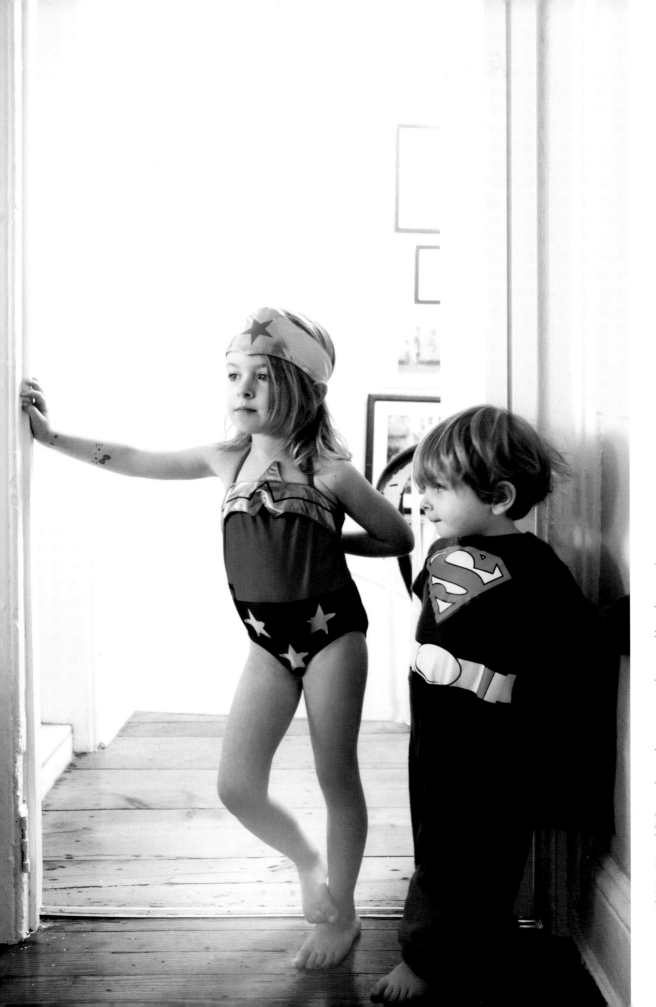

LEFT: Christina Hutson's little ones love to dress up as superheroes and have dance parties.

119

RIGHT: A love note written by Jade Berreau to her daughter Secret.

120

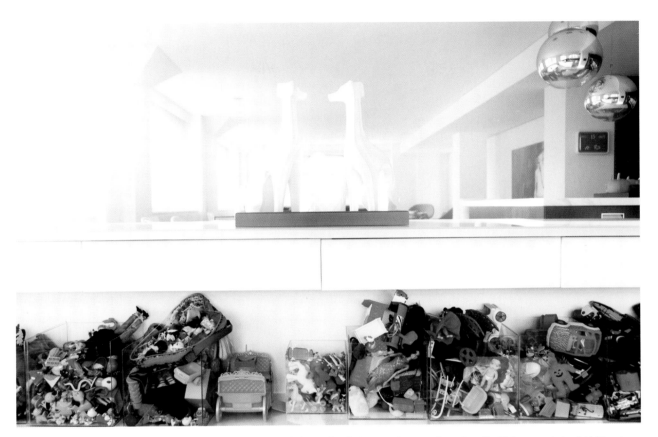

ABOVE: To maintain the minimal aesthetic of her downtown loft, jewelry designer and mom of two Jennifer Fisher corrals her kids' toys in sleek plastic bins. BELOW: Branding guru Ramya Giangola favors wooden toys for her daughter Chiara, such as this wood animal puzzle from Imagiplay.

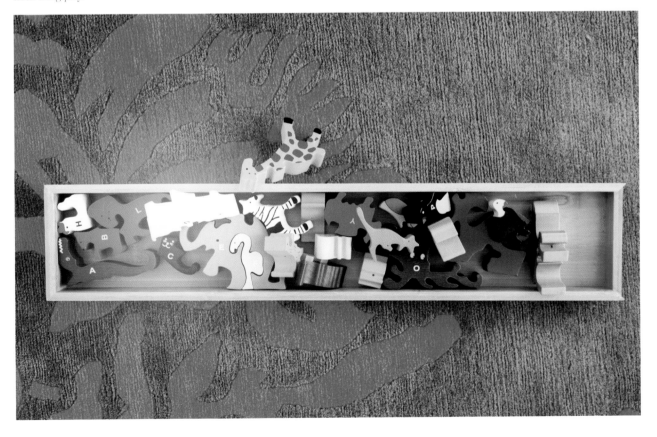

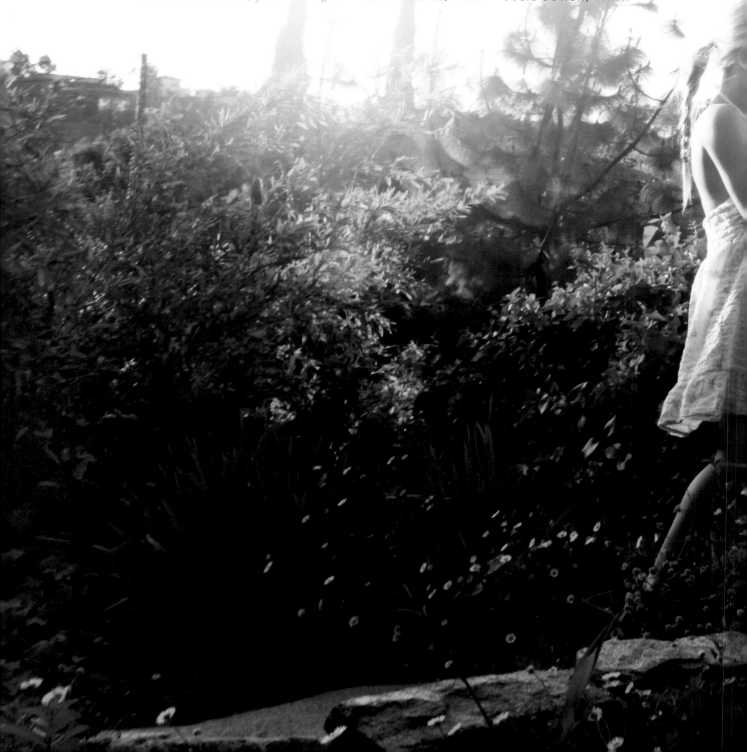

CHAPTER SIX

Glowing Beauty

JOSIE MARAN, *founder of Josie Maran Cosmetics* · JEANINE LOBELL, *makeup artist*

JEMIMA KIRKE, *artist & actress* · KATE YOUNG, *stylist* · PATI DUBROFF, *makeup artist*

MINNIE MORTIMER, *fashion designer* · KIRSTY HUME, *model* · JULIE BOWEN, *actress*

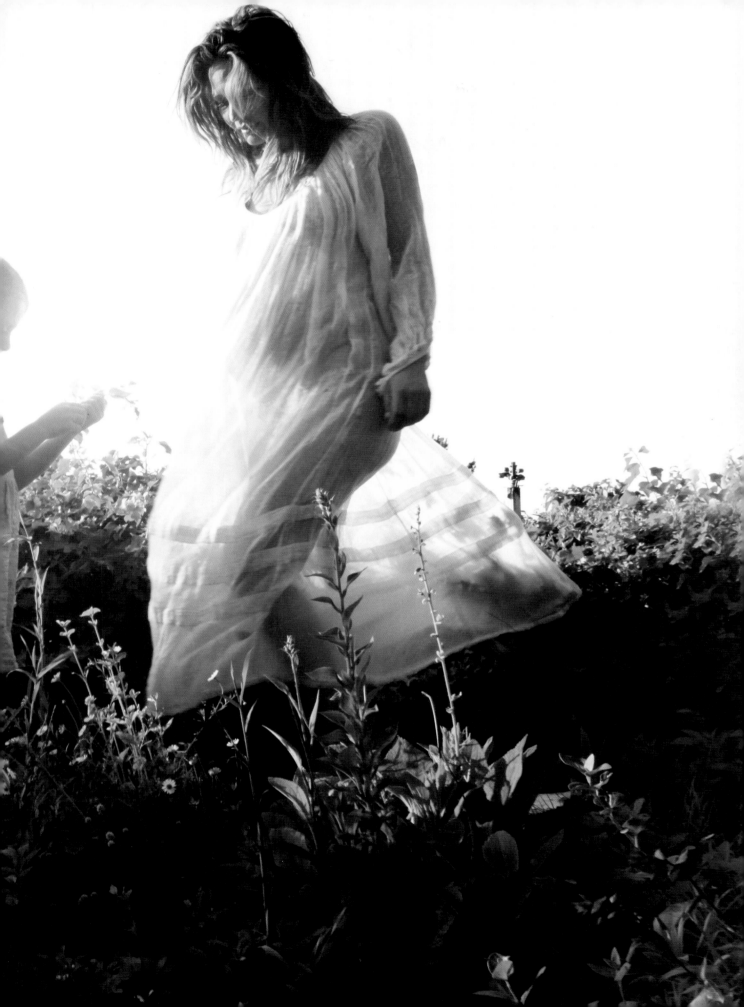

*I*n the words of model-turned-entrepreneur Josie Maran, any beauty product worth using since becoming a mom must be as hardworking as she is. Just as with motherhood, the mom of two believes that beauty is all about multitasking. Even before the baby arrives, it's time to take a step back and reevaluate.

For makeup artist Pati Dubroff, pregnancy was a time to go natural: "The skin is the largest organ and absorbs product—I wanted what I was putting on to be pure and nourishing to the pure being growing inside."

Maran, on the other hand, had a life-changing epiphany during her first pregnancy: She realized there was no "healthy makeup out there that was good enough for a makeup artist." True to her trailblazer spirit, she created it herself.

While most expectant moms will not take their desire for natural yet effective products to such great lengths, luckily for us all, the beauty mavens featured in this chapter have done the work for us. They've rounded up the best tips (honed over many years on film sets, fashion shoots, and around-the-world travels) for creating quick, easy, and healthy ways to feel beautiful.

As the mother of three daughters, legendary makeup artist Jeanine Lobell stresses the importance of focusing on inner beauty. She often repeats one simple sentiment to her girls: "It's not about the pretty." Determined to get them through their teenage years as unscathed as possible, Lobell works hard to "help them create a strong sense of self."

Here we explore beauty from the inside, including meditation (Jemima Kirke practiced a little every day throughout her pregnancies), must-have products (it's all about finding the perfect concealer), and tried-and-tested techniques—from alternatives to hairstyling without heat to showering with toddlers.

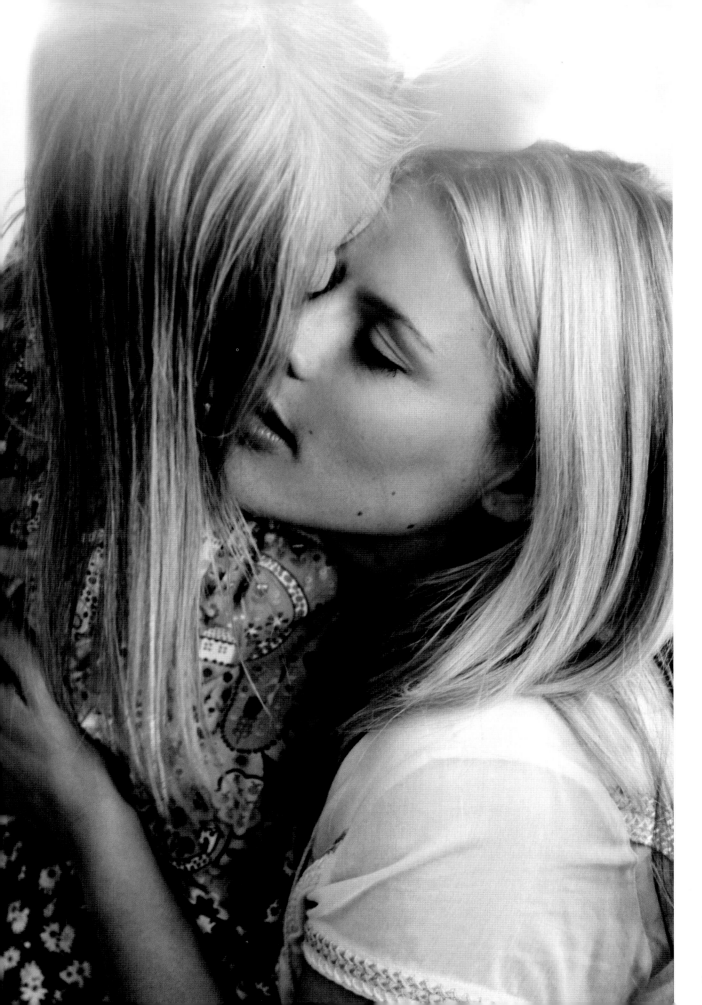

Josie MARAN

FOUNDER OF JOSIE MARAN COSMETICS

Daughter Rumi Joon,
photographed at five years old
(Josie was photographed at six months pregnant with daughter Indi)
Laurel Canyon, California

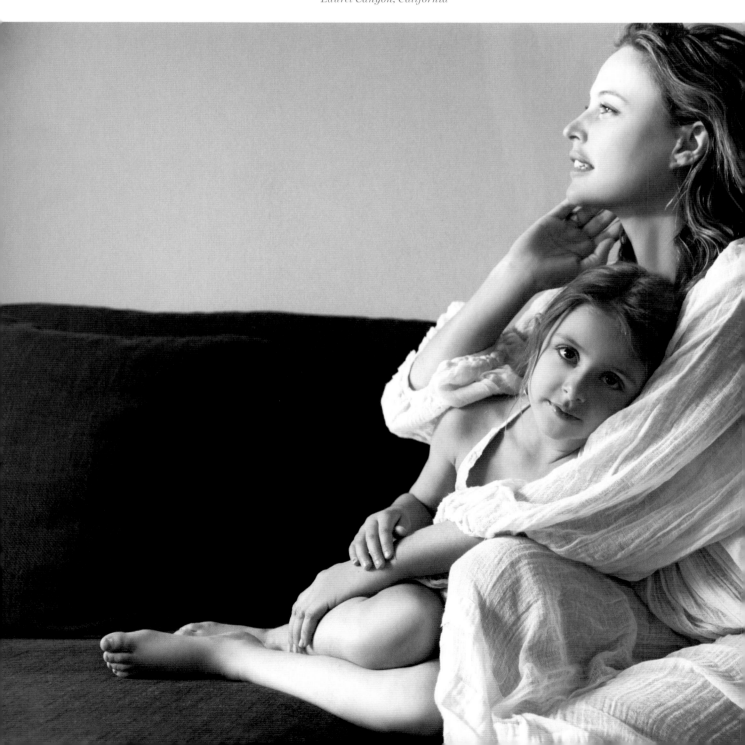

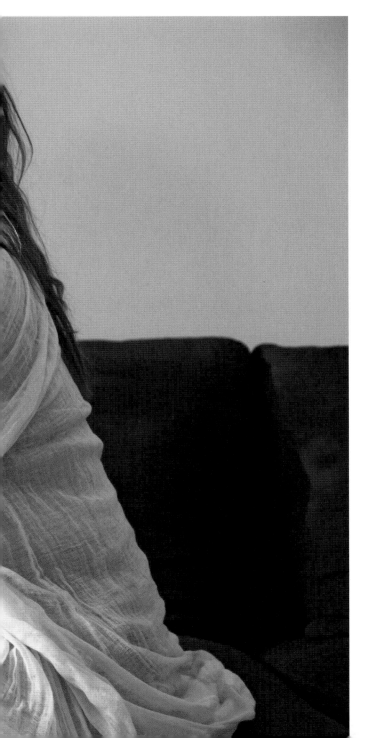

Josie Maran burst onto the modeling scene at the tender age of twelve and was working full-time by seventeen. Supermodel status followed, thanks to a decade-long Maybelline contract, countless magazine covers, and appearances in the iconic *Sports Illustrated* swimsuit issue. Little did the world know that Maran's biggest career accomplishments were still to come. While pregnant with her first child, the mom-to-be conceptualized her namesake line of eco-conscious, makeup-artist-approved product line. Six years later, Josie Maran Cosmetics has become the go-to eco-beauty brand. Maran's love of nature influences every aspect of her life—she delivered daughter Rumi in the lavender-filled field of their Laurel Canyon family compound. It's all about balance for this earth mother, though in some cases, Maran admits, extremes win out: "I'm either in four-inch heels or barefoot."

JOSIE ON MOTHERHOOD: I wish I was better at everything! Isn't that the essence of being a mom—trying to do everything better every day?

BEAUTY DURING PREGNANCY: I became obsessed with what I was putting on and in my body. That's when I discovered how toxic some beauty products are and how hard it is to find cosmetics that are top quality, luxurious, and healthy. I decided to create my own line of natural, effective beautifiers—for myself, and for every woman out there.

PREGNANCY MUST-HAVES: Argan oil is the best stretch-mark preventer in the world. And another added bonus is that once the baby is born, it is also a huge help with the baby's cradle cap.

BEAUTY AFTER BABY: I have four words for you: Downsize your beauty routine. After I gave birth to my first daughter, Rumi Joon, I barely had time to take a shower. I definitely didn't have time to try on new colors or even experimenting with a new mask or cream. I needed to know that my makeup worked and that it was good for me.

BEAUTY RULES: The most important beauty rule I can possibly impart to my daughters is simple: Love yourself. We actually make a ritual of it—we each say "I love you" to ourselves every day. I can see their faces soften and glow every time we do it. I also try to teach them to enjoy their beauty, and that less is more.

BEST ADVICE: When I had Rumi, my mom told me to remember how I was as a child. If you can be empathetic with your kid and see their perspective, you can always find a solution.

MY BEAUTY LOOK IS . . . Inspired, effortless, glowing.

Josie's Routine

* Argan oil as a booster in a favorite moisturizer or serum.
* My Matchmaker foundation. There are only three shades for the whole world, so it's super-easy.
* Then I use my Argan Color Stick for my lipstick, blush, and even for eye shadow—one product for my whole face.
* To get rid of under-eye bags, I refrigerate my Bear Naked Makeup Remover Wipes before putting them over my eyes.

TIME-SAVING TIPS:

* Multitaskers are my savior—products that I can use on my cheeks, lips, eyes, and even on my body.
* Techniques like using my fingers instead of brushes, which actually helps me get a better application.
* Braiding my hair overnight to get a beachy wave the next day.
* Carrying my Argan Infinity Cream with me at all times—I even use it to help soothe boo-boos on my two daughters.

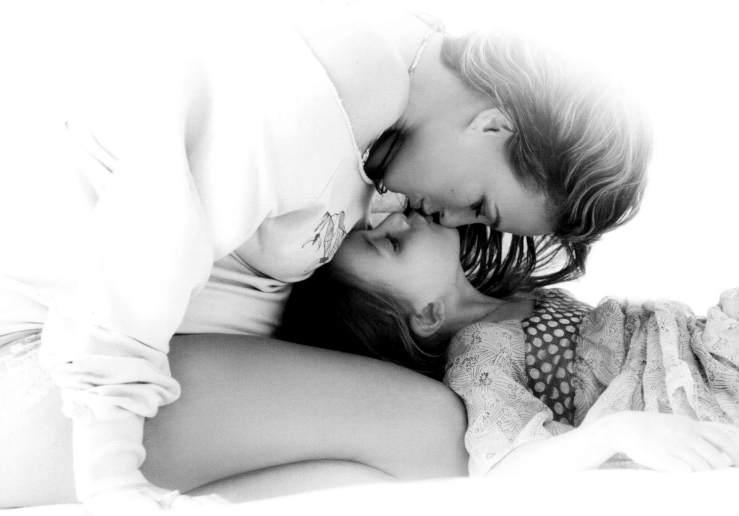

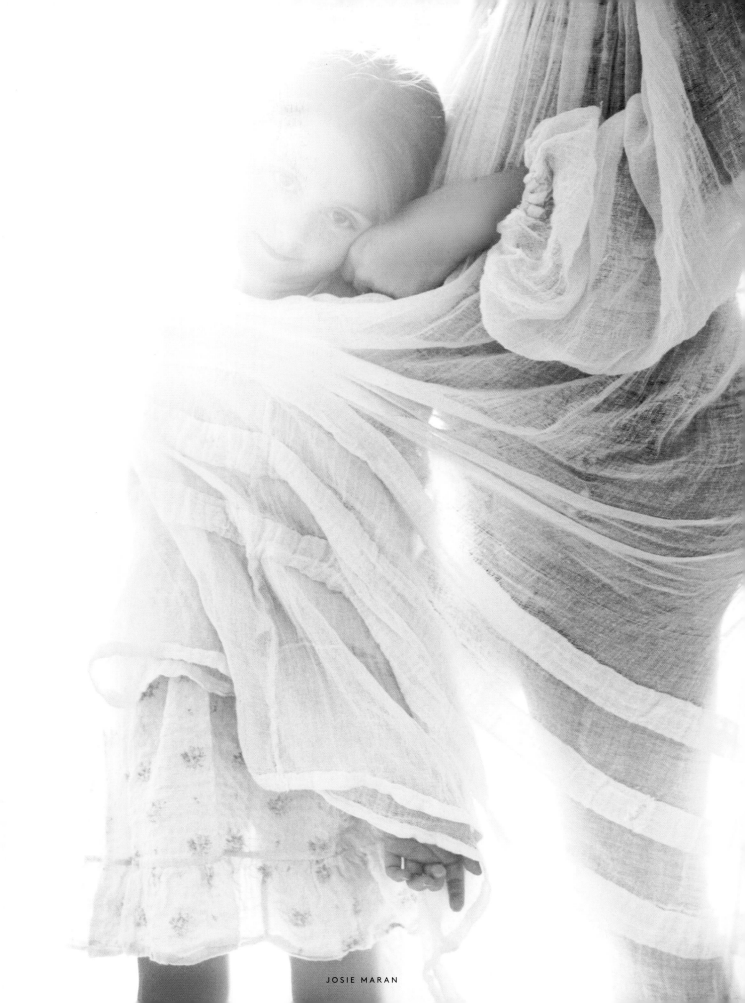

JOSIE MARAN

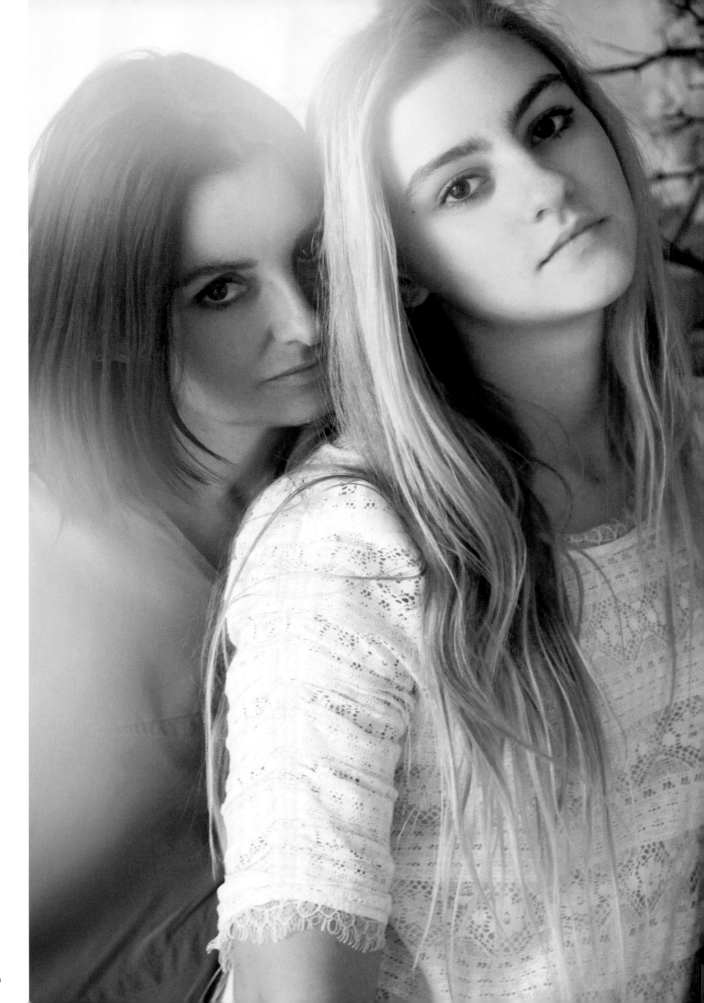

Jeanine LOBELL

MAKEUP ARTIST

———————————

Daughter Esme,
photographed at sixteen
(son Bailey, twenty years old, and daughters Wallis and Poppy,
thirteen and ten years old, respectively, seen on page 70)
New York, New York

With an illustrious career that spans two decades, makeup artist (and original Stila Cosmetics founder) Jeanine Lobell is a veritable beauty legend. Not only is she the mastermind behind iconic editorials from *Vogue* and *W*, she's also responsible for beautifying Natalie Portman, as well as a handful of other beautiful (and smart) mamas like Michelle Williams, Cate Blanchett, and Rachel Weisz. No surprise, then, that this mother of four is an endless stream of wisdom on everything from relationships (she's been happily married to actor Anthony Edwards for more than twenty years) to home décor. And, lucky for her, Lobell's beauty genius spills over into their time together.

JEANINE ON MOTHERHOOD: Once you have kids, everything naturally changes. It's supposed to. If you see change as something hard, it will be difficult. The key is not to see things as "challenges." The key to a long-lasting relationship is acceptance, laughter, self-reflection.

TIME-SAVING TIPS: A great haircut is key. The trick is finding someone who cuts your hair to the way it actually falls, so when it dries, you don't have to style it. I am a mascara and liner girl, but I always say, "Find the one thing about your face you think is great and the one thing you don't like—play up the one that is 'good,' learn to fix the problem, and ignore the rest." I live for mascara and a fuchsia or red lip.

Jeanine's Routine

* Chanel mascara
* SK-II face cream
* Klorane
* Eye patches for puffiness
* YSL Touche Eclat concealer: I would be a mess without it.

BEAUTY INDULGENCE: Every few months I get a Sapphire laser facial.

THE THIRTY-SECOND FACE: Giorgio Armani Lip Maestro: It's a liquid matte in a lip-gloss wand, which comes in oranges, reds, fuchsias. I throw that on, and I'm done.

FAVORITE BEAUTY LOOK: I feel the best with a tan and only mascara—I don't want to feel like I'm wearing a mask.

MOTHER-DAUGHTER BEAUTY RITUAL: We go to Jin Soon regularly for manis and pedis—they are the best!

BEAUTY RULES: Because of my job, my daughters really live and breathe beauty—whether it's in my makeup closets or visiting me at work, they are surrounded by it, so I teach them that it's not about the pretty. Being beautiful helps in life, for sure, but you cannot just be about that. With my girls, it's all about helping them create a strong sense of self. If they are really clear on who they are and what you expect and love about them, they will be able to get through their teen years much more easily.

BIGGEST SURPRISE: I love my kids so much it actually hurts.

MY BEAUTY LOOK IS . . . Easy, understated, slept in.

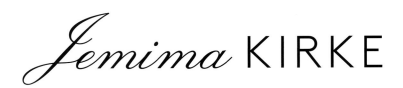

Jemima KIRKE

ARTIST & ACTRESS

Daughter Rafaella,
photographed at one year old
Brooklyn, New York

When London-born, New York–raised artist Jemima Kirke decided to have a child, she wondered how easily motherhood and creativity could coexist. Now a proud mother of two, Kirke is proving that her passions can mesh peacefully. The Brooklyn Heights home she shares with her husband has a decidedly romantic feel; vintage treasures fill the eclectic space, while a beguiling mix of art—from Robert Mapplethorpe to Alfred Wertheimer— covers the walls. As the now-infamous story reads, Kirke went from RISD-trained painter to accidental actress when filmmaker Lena Dunham, her childhood friend, persuaded her to star in her indie hit film *Tiny Furniture* as well as the highly obsessed–over HBO series *Girls*. Her character, Jessa, has quickly become a poster child of sorts for free-spirited, adventurous women everywhere. Artist, actress, mother, wife—Kirke deftly moves among roles with effortless charm.

JEMIMA ON MOTHERHOOD: When I found out I was having a baby, I wondered whether there were any success- ful female painters with children. When I actually asked the question, I realized there were a lot. I was worried about how I was going to do it. When I was younger, painting was something that was quite impulsive or even compulsive for me. When you're a mother, there's no room to be impulsive or compulsive—or it's better if you're not. I asked myself, "What am I going to lose by having a child?" And so far the answer is "nothing."

HARDEST PART: There's no more getting up and going somewhere because you've suddenly decided it would be fun—no impulsive actions, no last-minute trips or outings. Almost every action or trip must be thought out in ad- vance—seeing a movie, going out to dinner, taking a nap, walking the dog.

BEST ADVICE: Allow someone else to take care of your baby sometimes. It's good for them. It's good for you.

BEAUTY DURING PREGNANCY: I meditated a little every day and drank a ton of water (mainly because I was

always crazy thirsty). I also craved baths at weird hours, like four a.m. when I couldn't sleep, or first thing in the morn- ing. I just wanted to sit in the hot water and feel totally private, even if it was just for five minutes.

TIME-SAVING TIPS: When you become a mom, you really have to adapt your morning routine and rituals—they've got to be quick and efficient. I boiled down the whole skin-care routine to two things: Cetaphil (three seconds) and La Mer cream. It's super-expensive, but when I finally realized how to use it correctly, one jar would last me a year.

MOTHER-DAUGHTER BEAUTY: We love to paint on each other: markers, stickers, stamps, etc. If I go out at night, before I leave the house, I always kiss her hand and leave a lipstick mark. It seems to make her feel better about my leaving.

BEAUTY RULES: I like to point out something pretty or nice about her friends and people we meet, like their generos- ity or even just their lovely dress. That way, she might look for things to admire in people. She's always pointing at someone's hair or shoes and saying, "It's peedy!" or, "She a pincess!"

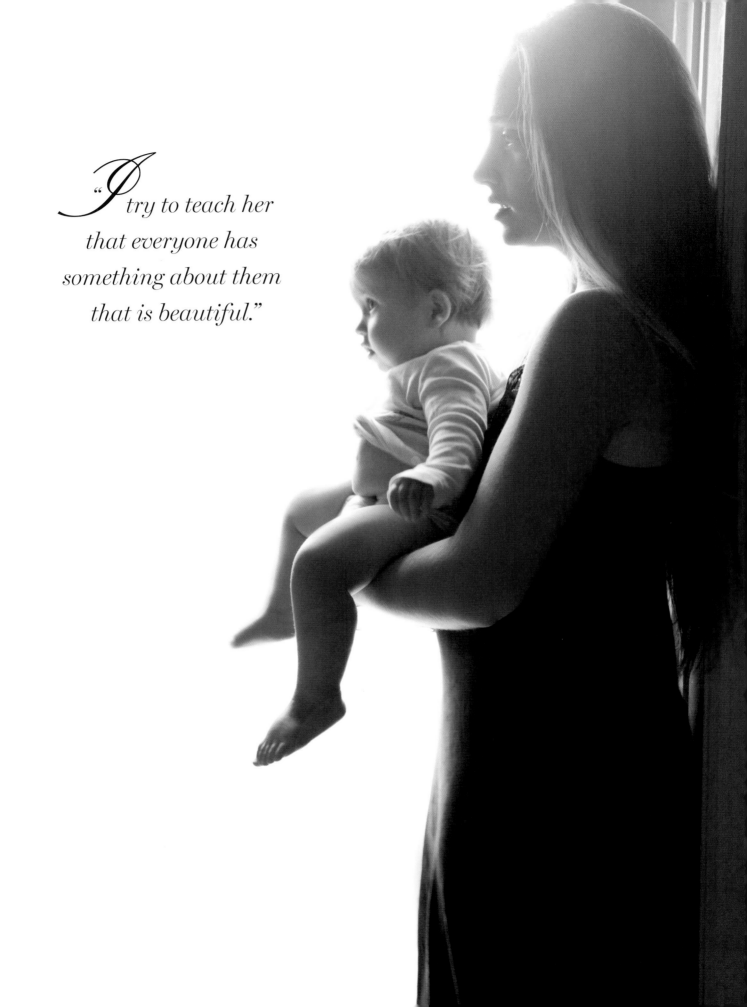

*"I try to teach her
that everyone has
something about them
that is beautiful."*

Kate YOUNG

STYLIST

Son Stellan, photographed at four years old
(not pictured: son Leif, age twenty months, seen on page 67)
Brooklyn, New York

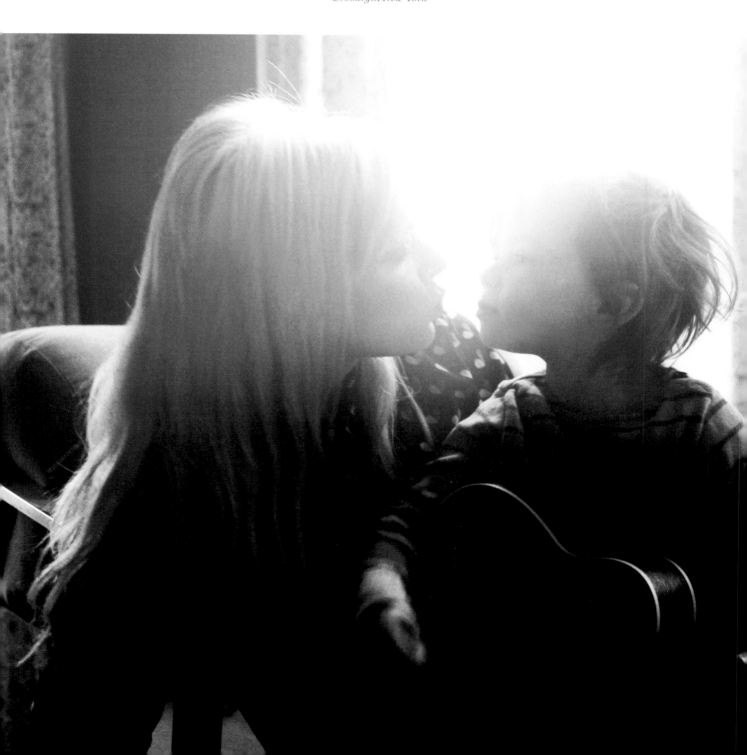

Kate Young has been called the most powerful stylist in Hollywood, but in her tight-knit Brooklyn neighborhood she's better known as Stellan and Leif's mom. After seven years at *Vogue*, where she started out as Anna Wintour's assistant, Young branched out on her own, and the rest, as they say, is history. From dressing her clients (and friends) Natalie Portman and Michelle Williams to designing her very own line for Target, Young is among the industry's most sought-after talents. Her own edgy-meets-classic wardrobe and signature "no makeup" makeup look achieve that hard-to-come-by combination of effortlessness and chic. Same goes for the eclectic pieces scattered around her boys' shared bedroom—from animal costumes and wood guitars to the impossibly cool tweed teddy bear given to her older son as a birth gift by the house of Chanel.

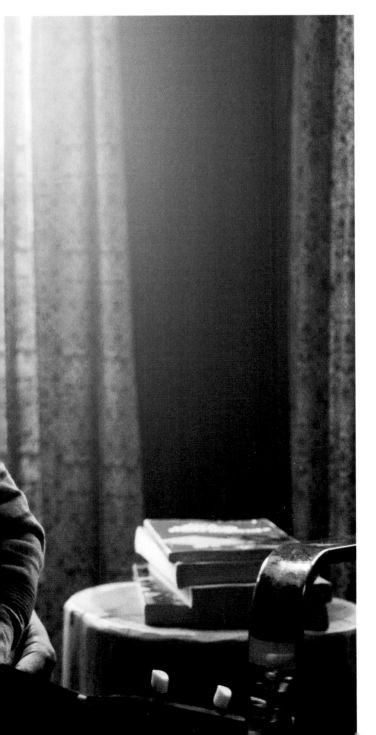

KATE ON MOTHERHOOD: I'm amazed by the village of people who help us raise these kids—my parents, my husband's parents, our nanny, the school, all of our friends. It blows my mind how incredible everyone is and how much they make up the fabric of the kids' lives.

BEST PART: As a mom, you get to experience what falling in love feels like again with each child.

HARDEST PART: It's all much harder with two kids and yet there's much less stress about the little one. I don't worry about Leif—his health, his development—I trust the process of him growing much more and he's a more laid-back little guy because of it. But chaos reigns now. With one I still felt like the house and my life were orderly. That is no longer the case.

BEST ADVICE: The advice given to me by every good mother I know is to trust my own instincts.

BEAUTY DURING PREGNANCY: I became very conscious about switching to more-natural products. I started using Weleda cleanser and Rodin oil when I first got pregnant—they work for me, and I continue to use them to this day. I also did tons of yoga with Mia at Lila Yoga and fell in love with their Mother's Special Blend Oil.

BEAUTY AFTER BABY: I can get showered and dressed in under ten minutes now. I don't wear makeup unless I'm going somewhere fancy, and then red lipstick makes me look pulled together in five seconds. Instead of blow-drying my hair, I just twist it and put it up with Odile Gilbert pins, and it dries straight with a good wave.

BEAUTY INDULGENCE: Facials with Joanna Vargas

MY BEAUTY LOOK IS . . . Super-blond.

Pati DUBROFF

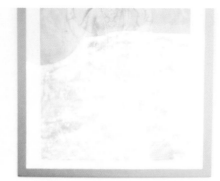

MAKEUP ARTIST

Daughter Bianca,
photographed at nine years old
Los Angeles, California

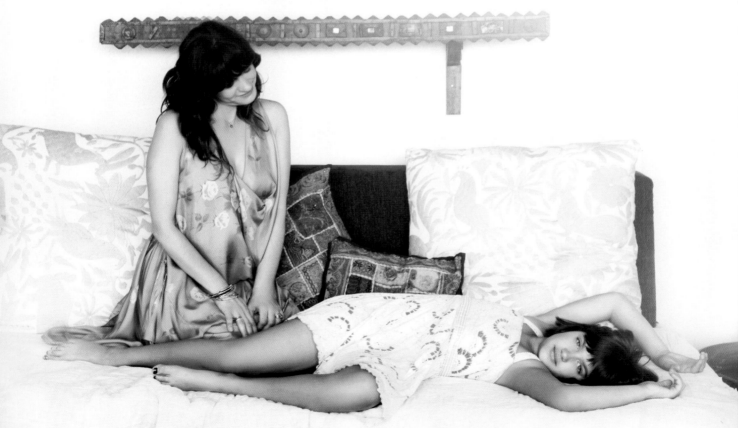

Pati Dubroff has the kind of career most makeup artists only dream of. After assisting the legendary François Nars, she branched off on her own, creating editorials for *Vogue*, *Vanity Fair*, and *Allure*, eventually snagging the coveted role of spokesperson for Dior and, later, Clarins. When she's not traveling the world with one of her devoted clients (including fellow moms Gwyneth Paltrow, Julianne Moore, and Charlize Theron), she's spending time high up in the Hollywood Hills with her trilingual daughter and Italian husband. Their calm oasis is filled with treasured objects found on their travels to Morocco and India, while plenty of outdoor space ensures that this close-knit family of three (plus a blue-eyed cat named Raja) feels worlds away from the hectic buzz of Los Angeles. Much like her accomplished mom, nine-year-old Bianca is already a prolific painter, fluent in three languages, and, not surprisingly, loves a good lip gloss.

BEAUTY DURING PREGNANCY: I became very aware of what I was putting on my skin. The skin is the largest organ and absorbs product—I wanted what I was putting on to be pure and nourishing to the pure being growing inside. I started to look for products that are free of all synthetics, ones that generally were created by fellow women who are aware of the preciousness of the body. I continue to focus on products like this now. Being pregnant gave me the gift of awareness!

PREGNANCY ROUTINE: Baths, for me, were essential. During pregnancy, my senses seemed to be heightened, so anything with synthetic fragrances made me feel sick. I wanted things that were soft and natural, like lavender oil and pure coconut oil, which I used as a body moisturizer and to prevent stretch marks.

BEAUTY AFTER BABY: I definitely had to scale back on beautification time after having my daughter. I don't wear a lot of makeup day to day (if any!) but definitely found I didn't have time to "do" my hair as much. Wash and go is where it's at now.

Pati's Routine

* Kevyn Aucoin lash curler to wake up my eyes
* Dry shampoo for the many days my roots need some help
* Rita Hazan Root Concealer to hide the grays when I have no time to go see my colorist
* John Masters Organics Sea Mist sea salt spray with lavender

TIME-SAVING TIPS
Skin: It's all about multitasking. If I'm going to do a mask, I have to jam it in at the end of my bath. No more lounging around with beauty products—it's all about taking advantage of time when it becomes available.
Hair: I use a sea salt spray to get fast beachy waves without relying on curling irons. Sometimes, when my hair is still wet, I twist my hair into little "Princess Leia" buns to enhance the curl without having to use heat.

BEAUTY INDULGENCE: I try to make the time to get facials and hair color, but I tend to wait until it's a dire need as opposed to staying on top of regular maintenance. I love the idea of occasionally getting pampered, but I find I'm more drawn toward getting much-needed massages instead of more "fluff" treatments.

MOTHER-DAUGHTER BEAUTY: We love to take baths together, and thankfully we have a very large tub, so we still fit. Bath time is when we talk about our day, catch up, and reconnect.

BEAUTY RULES: I really want her to understand that beauty encompasses so many elements. Sadly, our society is fixated on the exterior when describing beauty. I try to instill in her the awareness that beauty lies in the spirit, the soul of each person. It's not about looks, but rather how you live in this world, how you treat other people. I remind her that the true beauties I have met are the ones who have the most beautiful spirits. Also, healthy is what is beautiful. Confidence is beautiful.

MY BEAUTY LOOK IS . . . Easygoing, natural, effortless.

Minnie MORTIMER

FASHION DESIGNER

Daughter Tuesday,
photographed at four years old
Los Angeles, California

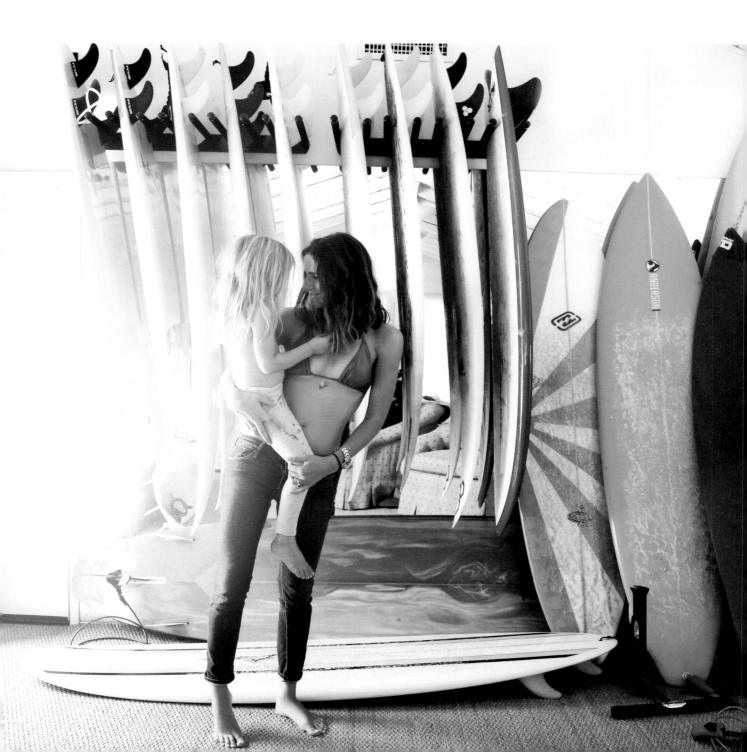

Designer Minnie Mortimer may be a born-and-bred New Yorker at heart, but her spirit is pure California sunshine. After meeting and falling in love with Oscar-winning screenwriter Stephen Gaghan, Mortimer made the move cross-country and has embraced her new Los Angeles life with giddy enthusiasm. As she is an avid surfer, the salt air and ocean waves affect everything from her style—think striped minidresses from her namesake line worn with easy-to-slip-on Isabel Marant boots—to her tousled beauty look.

MINNIE ON MOTHERHOOD: It just keeps getting better and better. I keep thinking, OK, now this is my favorite age; it can't get any better than this, but it does!

BEST PART: The pure, unfiltered, unconditional love and joy that can only come from children and animals.

TREASURED ROUTINE: Eating dinner as a family every night. You don't need to cook, but set the table, sit down at the same time and get up at the same time.

BEAUTY DURING PREGNANCY: I switched to all non-toxic products. My favorites were cocoa butter (and lots of it) and Deborah Lippmann nontoxic nail polish.

BEAUTY RULES: I try to teach her to take care of her body and be gentle with it.

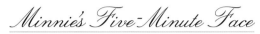

Minnie's Five-Minute Face

★ Aquaphor
★ YSL mascara
★ Laura Mercier tinted moisturizer
★ Stila cheek stain

TIME-SAVING TIPS & TRICKS: I use wipes for everything! As makeup removers, to get stains out of my clothes, to clean my hands, the steering wheel, even the table at a café.

BEAUTY INDULGENCE: Massage—I am addicted. And I love having my hair done for me at Drybar.

MY BEAUTY LOOK IS . . . Minimal, fresh, summery.

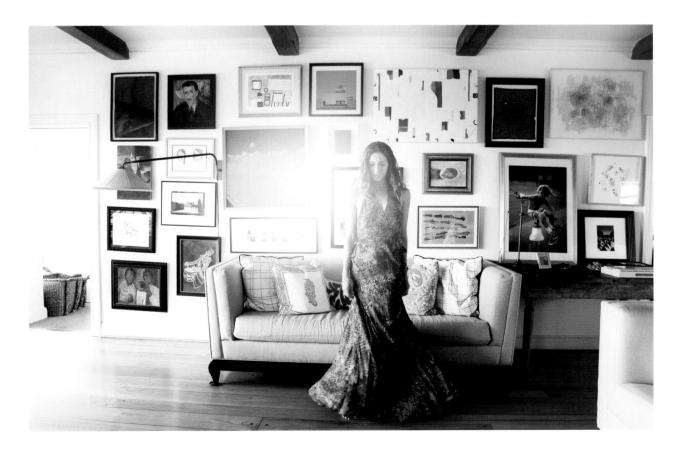

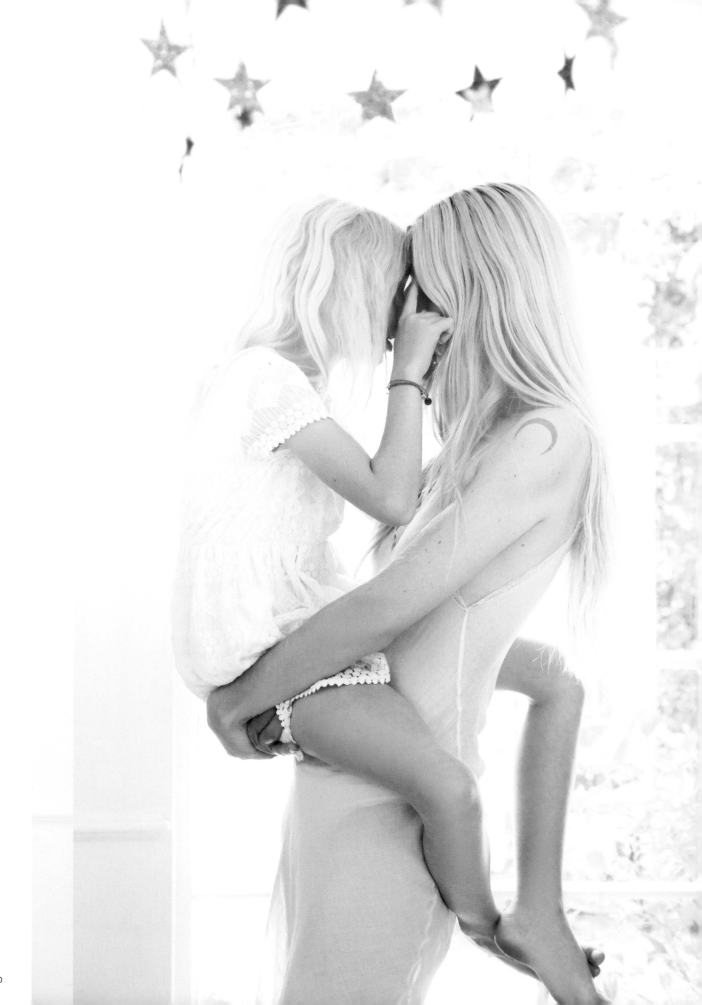

Kirsty HUME

MODEL

Daughter Violet,
photographed at ten years old
Los Angeles, California

In stark contrast to her busy life as an in-demand model for the past two decades, Kirsty Hume's peaceful Los Angeles home feels millions of miles away from the buzzing fashion world—and that's exactly how she likes it. The tranquil world she's created for her ten-year-old daughter is filled with plenty of arts and crafts, and quality time with their pet rabbit. Mother and daughter are beautifully in sync as they move through life as a close-knit duo—whether they're cooking, knitting, or having one of their nightly dance parties.

KIRSTY ON MOTHERHOOD: I try to plan ahead as much as possible, to make large one-pot meals that will last a few days, and I always remind myself that it takes a village!

LIFE LESSONS: I want my daughter to know that every action we take ripples out into this world. And she must always listen to herself, to that little voice inside that knows.

BEST PART: Cuddling with her, getting little notes that say "I love you" all the time, and watching her grow up!

BEAUTY DURING PREGNANCY: I rubbed oil onto my belly religiously every day, and got pregnancy massages.

TIME-SAVING TIPS: Less is more: Just use a little concealer where needed instead of a full base. I feel sexiest when I'm fairly natural—a touch of concealer and blush.

MOTHER-DAUGHTER BEAUTY: Violet will often moisturize with me after taking a bath or shower, and she likes it when I give her little mini massages.

BEAUTY RULES: I try to teach her to love herself as she is.

MY BEAUTY LOOK IS . . . Very natural!

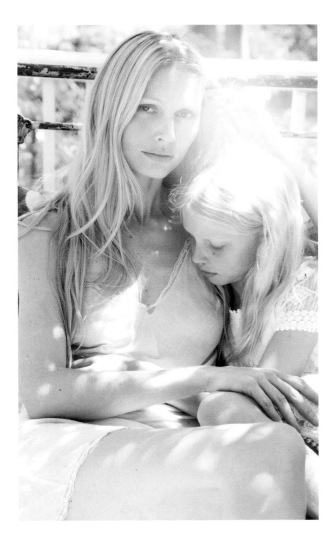

Julie BOWEN

ACTRESS

Twins Gustav and John and son Oliver,
photographed at four and six years old, respectively
Los Angeles, California

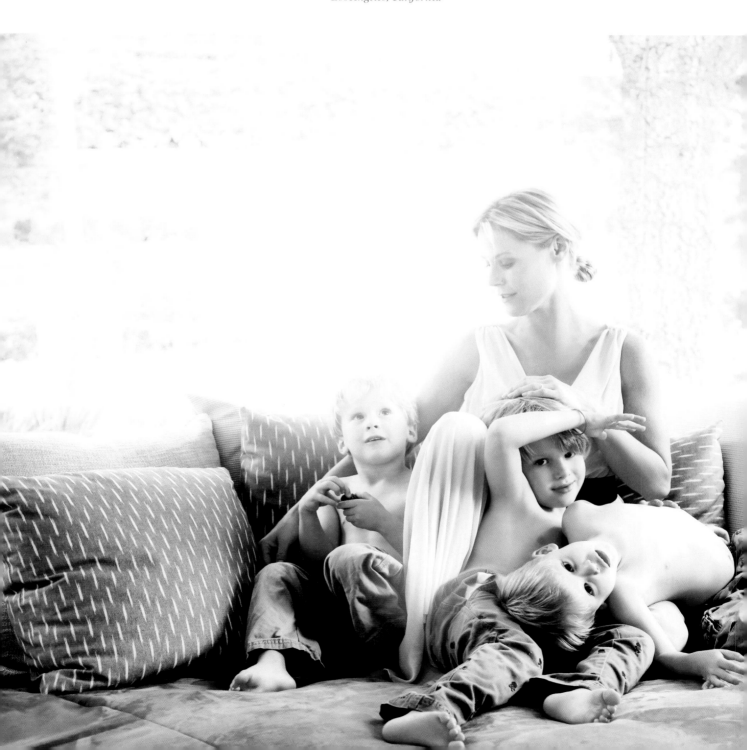

At first glance, the similarities between actress Julie Bowen and her TV alter ego, Claire Dunphy on America's favorite sitcom *Modern Family*, seem uncanny. Both have three children, lots of energy, and a dry, sarcastic wit. Spending time with the real-life supermom, however, it quickly becomes clear that the similarities end there. While Claire's approach to motherhood errs on the side of overbearing, Julie's MO is much more mellow. In her elegant yet laid-back Los Angeles home, she finds true happiness in being a mom to her rambunctious, blond-haired beauties. With her hectic work schedule, it's no surprise that Bowen's approach to beauty is all about ease and speed—spending time with her boys wins out over pampering any day. The result? Manicures and pedicures fall by the wayside in favor of digging in the dirt and jumping in the pool. For Bowen, being a mom is quite simply "what it's all about."

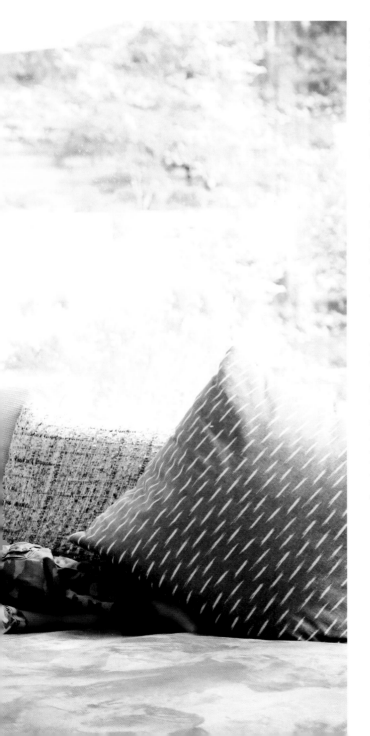

JULIE ON MOTHERHOOD: I am deeply involved with my kids, which gives me less time to be deeply involved in me. That's OK. I was deeply involved in me for three decades, and the end result was . . . eh. I didn't cure cancer or write the great American novel. I am happy to have these little people who demand so much, even though it means that in some areas my quality of life (sleep, food, hair color) is diminished.

BEST PART: They are pure joy and pure challenge all the time. There is no balance. There is only the next crisis in front of me. When there is no crisis, I try to take a mental picture to file away and think, "This is good. This is what it's all about. It will never be better than this moment." Then one of them stomps on my hand or bludgeons the other with a stick, and it's back to crisis mode.

HARDEST PART: Being a mom is hard because I say no a hundred times a day. Sometimes I think keeping my three boys alive means trading in my sense of humor for a drill sergeant's vigilance. I love them so much it actually hurts to be so relentlessly bossy, but honestly, my kids try to kill each other every day. (Let's start the car! Let's do a flip on the sidewalk! Let's throw hard, pointy objects at each other's heads!). Still, at least once a day, they break my heart with their "Mama, Mama, Mama!" and hands gripping my legs and tears over skinned knees or someone not sharing.

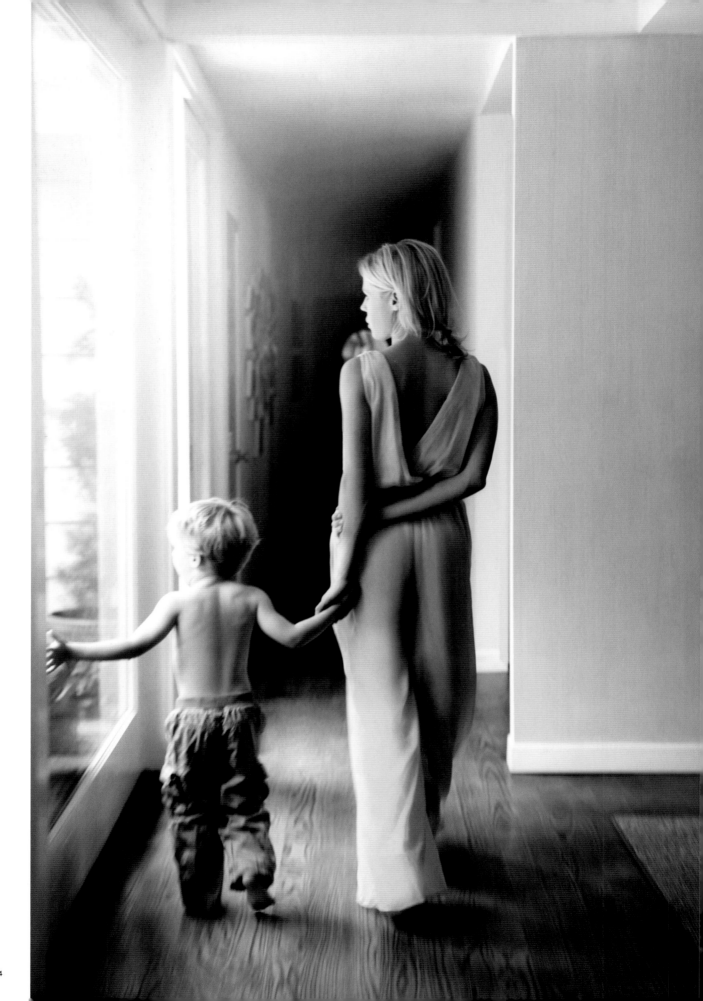

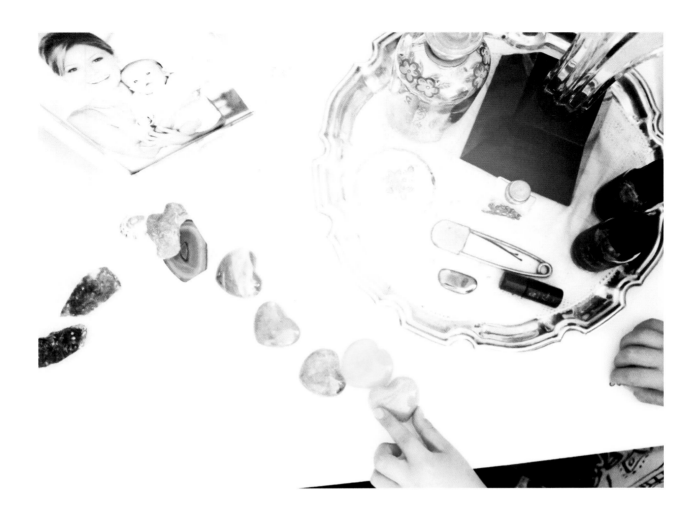

BEAUTY FROM WITHIN: I don't drink enough water. I hate it. I have to force myself to swallow plain water like it's a punishment. I like Fresca. And I like black coffee. I make myself drink green tea every day, but it's medicine to me. Food is just a fuel source, and many days I may as well eat a cardboard capsule full of "food nutrients" like Judy Jetson. Every now and again I sit down to a proper meal, but it's disconcertingly rare. I eat cold waffles and tepid broccoli off my children's plates.

MY BEAUTY LOOK IS . . . I've had the benefit of beautiful photography to make me look good in a picture while the reality is I am over forty, at times exhausted, and frequently fall asleep on the couch with a full face of makeup! I have endless beauty indulgences whenever I am working. Every time I get ready for work or a work event, I have a team of professionals dressing, drying, glossing . . . That is work mode. It's lovely. Home mode is chlorine-soaked hair and discovering that A&D diaper ointment is a passable moisturizer in a pinch. I haven't had a manicure on my own steam in over a year. I don't care a bit. If I need one for work, I'll get it, but otherwise, screw it. I have been known to paint only the one toenail peeking out of a peep-toe Louboutin before an event rather than spend an hour at a nail salon. It's not perfect, it's not classy, but I don't care. I'm imperfect as hell.

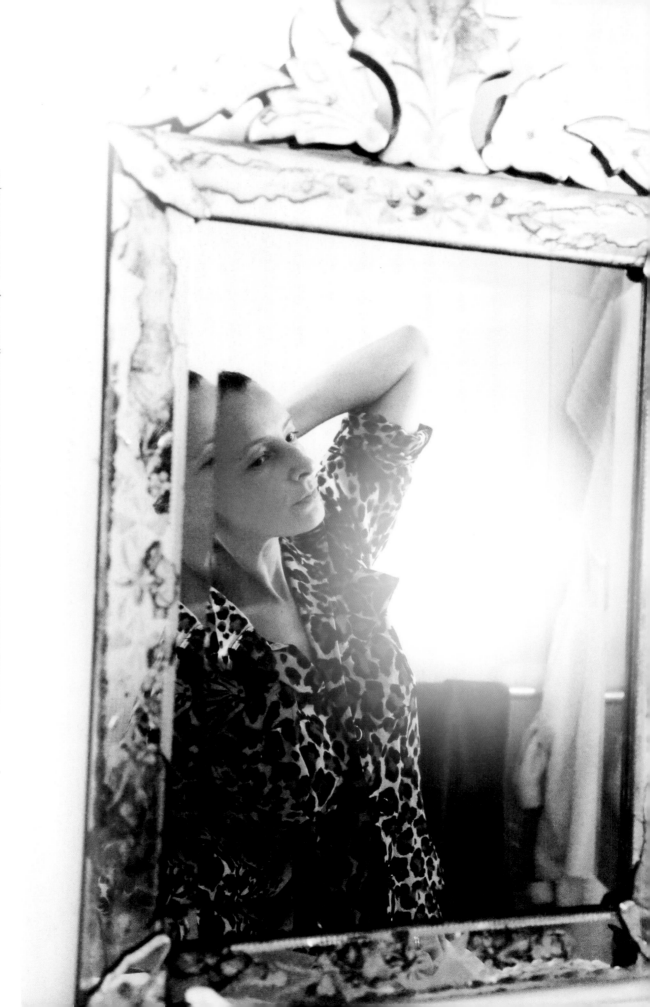

RIGHT: "I use oil all the time—Christophe Robin lavender for hair, Sultane de Saba carrot and rose for face, and Santa Maria Novella Melograno for body." –*Caroline Deroche Pasquier*

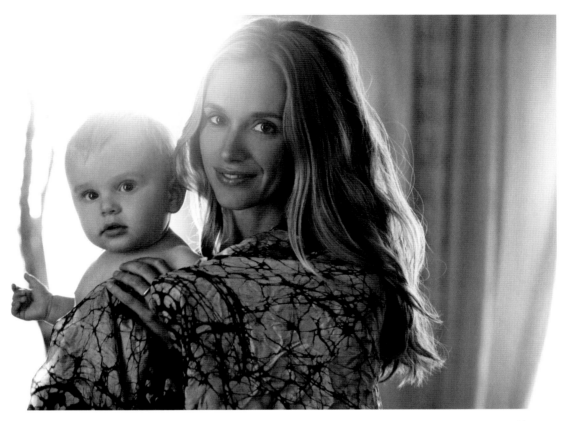

ABOVE: "I can get by with four makeup products: a light powder, Bare Minerals bronzer, Buxom Lash mascara, and Burt's Bees tinted lip balm. And I am obsessed with the Tata Harper skincare line. To save time, and for a little marital bonding, my husband cuts my hair." *–Rachelle Hruska* BELOW: "I don't blow-dry my hair, which is a major time saver. I just use a little Moroccan hair oil. For my skin, I use Colbert MD skincare products, which help to conceal all my sleepless nights." *–Jeanann Williams*

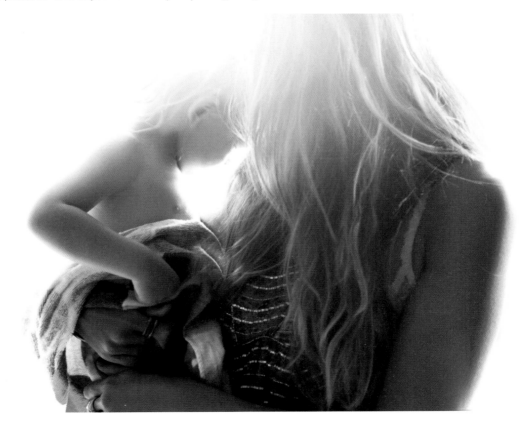

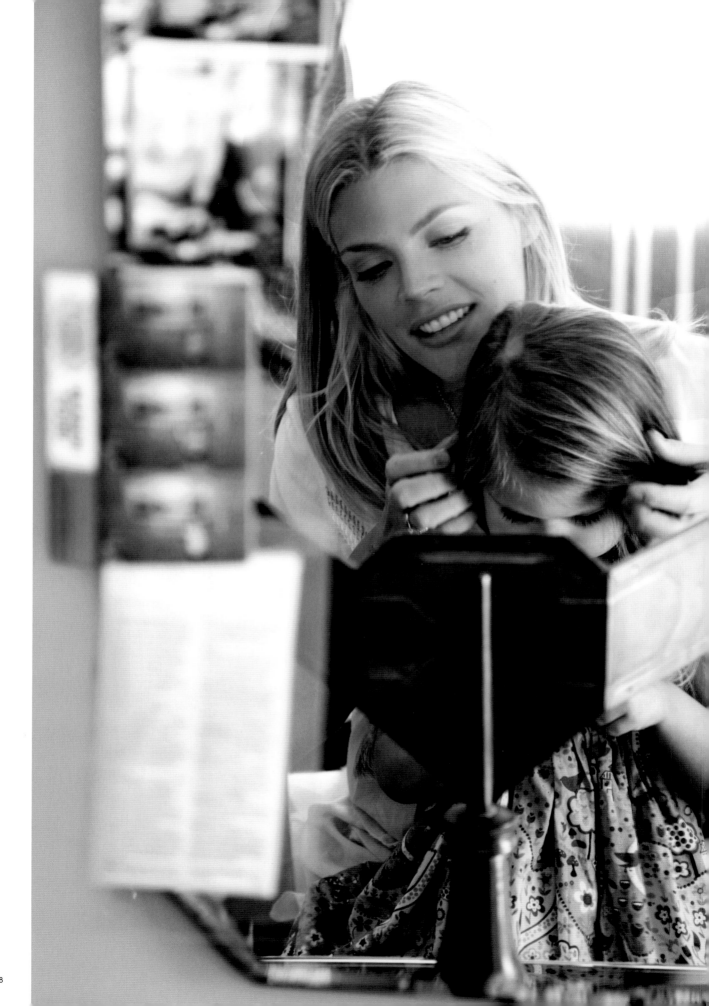

"When I have no time to get ready, I just put on lip balm, sunscreen, and braid my hair, then wrap it on top of my head (great for when your hair's a little dirty)."

—BUSY PHILIPPS, *actress*

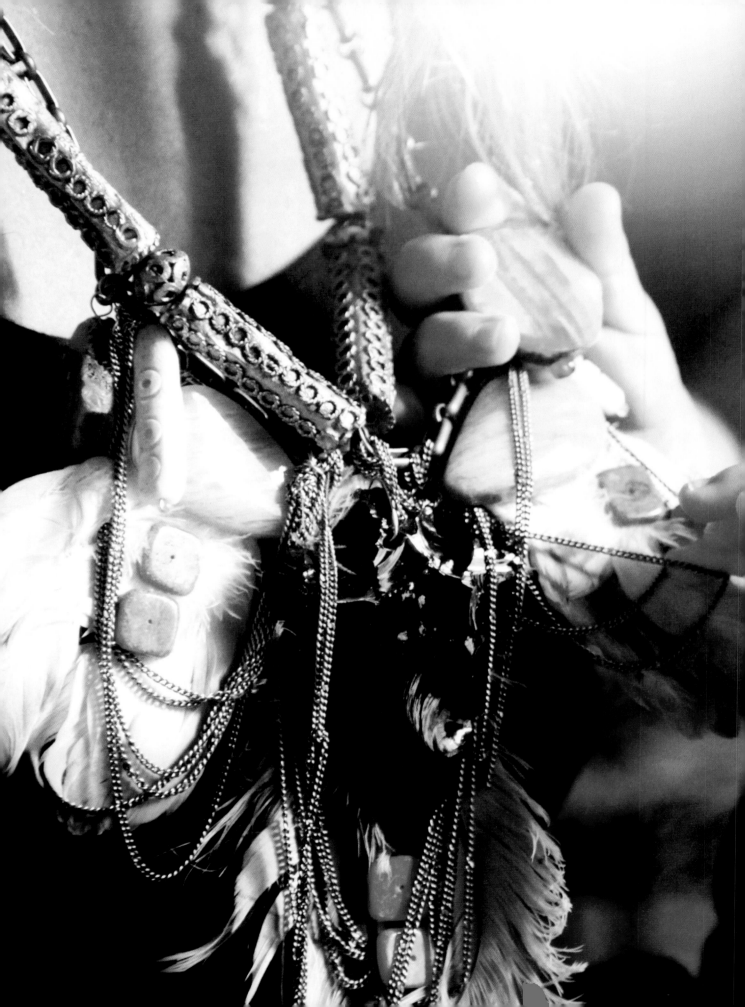

CHAPTER SEVEN

Style Sense

SELMA BLAIR, *actress* · CAROLINE DEROCHE PASQUIER, *Givenchy international public relations director*

JENNIFER FISHER, *jewelry designer* · YASMIN SEWELL, *fashion consultant*

MEREDITH KAHN, *jewelry designer* · JUNE AMBROSE, *stylist* · SARA BLAKELY, *Spanx founder*

*F*or most women, the transition into mom mode means a natural evolution of their personal style. The first phase of the transformation involves a steep learning curve—all of a sudden, you're dressing around a widened midsection, but the cute little bump is nowhere in sight. The biggest surprise for me was that my belly didn't go from flat to full-on baby bump overnight. The first five months felt like I was in limbo—my waistline was expanding, but the belly was not protruding enough to actually show it off. During this time, the key was to maintain my personal style—that meant skinny jeans, oversize silk blouses, and heels (always heels).

For jewelry designer Meredith Kahn, pregnancy was a time to adapt her edgy yet feminine style to her rapidly changing silhouette. Her first order of business: "I took the skinny waistband off my leather leggings and replaced it with a wider band to make them into maternity pants." This quick fix is a style—and money—saver. Her style advice for moms-to-be is simple: "If leather pants are your thing, and you're afraid you can't do it anymore once you get pregnant and become a mom, just adjust them." And, she admits, leather has the added bonus of holding you in a little. Once the bump becomes prominent, Kahn's approach is to embrace it. "It's OK once you're into your second trimester to really work the curves. A hint of cleavage is really sexy on a pregnant woman. Try to get into the earth mother look—it doesn't last, so enjoy it while it does."

As the next phase, new motherhood, begins, the focus shifts to function and how to seamlessly meld your "look"—whether that's ultra-feminine, minimal, or classic—with your new role. Spanx founder, and mama to an active three-year-old, Sara Blakely has traded in her stilettos for sneakers, and admits that she's been happy to embrace a more "casual and comfortable style."

While their personal style may vary, one thing each of the moms featured in this chapter can agree on is that creating a uniform of sorts is essential. Start with the basics—tailored tees (comfy and polished-looking), figure-flattering jeans, and a basic blazer—add versatile ankle boots (with a sturdy heel) plus a mix of jewelry, and go from there. Layer in personal touches, like prints, pops of color, and vintage elements, to make the look match your mood. For these seven trendsetters, motherhood has only enhanced their style, allowing them to grow and experiment. Each has cultivated the powerful confidence that comes with motherhood to let her true personality shine through.

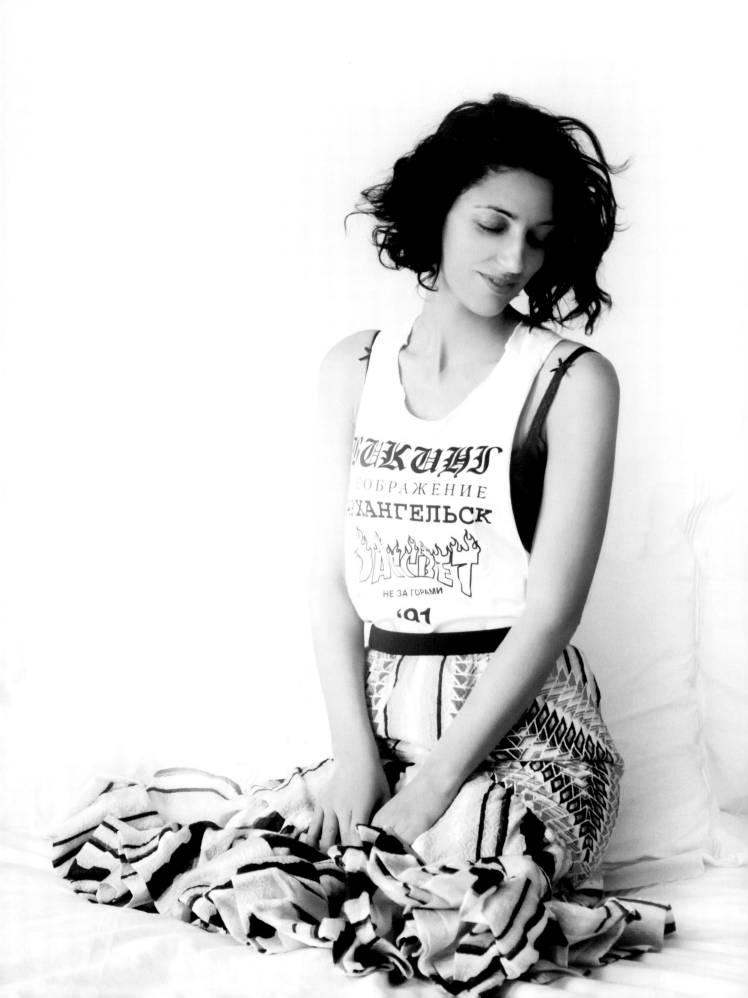

Selma BLAIR

ACTRESS

Son Arthur,
photographed at eighteen months old
Los Angeles, California

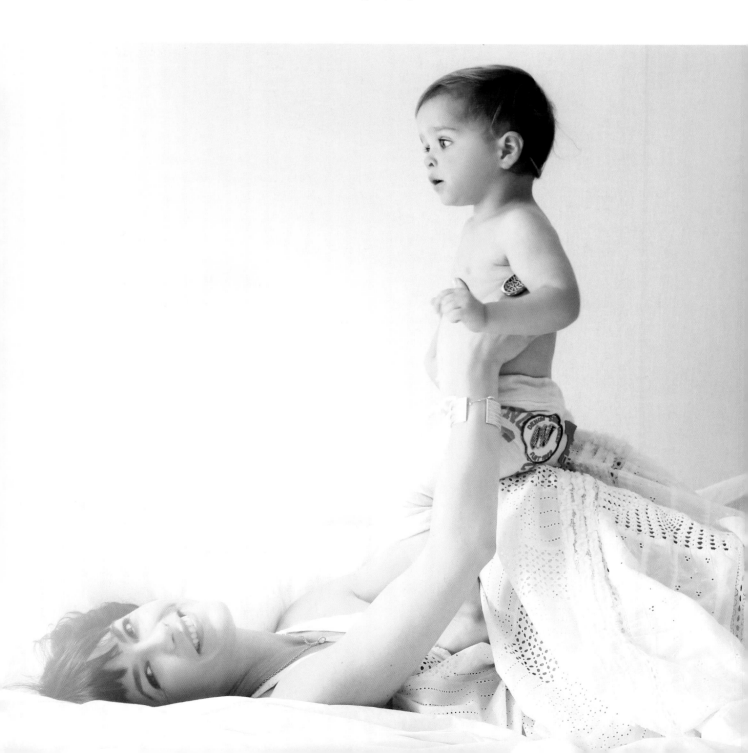

For actress Selma Blair, motherhood has turned the world as she knew it upside down in the most wonderful ways imaginable. The birth of her son, Arthur, in 2011 transformed this fashion darling into someone who can no longer even look at black clothing ("I'm just too happy for it", she admits). She's even learned to embrace pink, the color her son loves to see her in the most. As a working mom, Blair has managed to take a step back and embrace the benefits of balancing her career with life as a single mom. "If he sees that I'm happy and strong . . . then that is the best thing for him." With her busy schedule, downtime with Arthur is sacred. "I never thought I'd be one of those people who cherish every second," she admits. "I don't think any other miracle could have grounded me in this way—I appreciate every second I'm in his company."

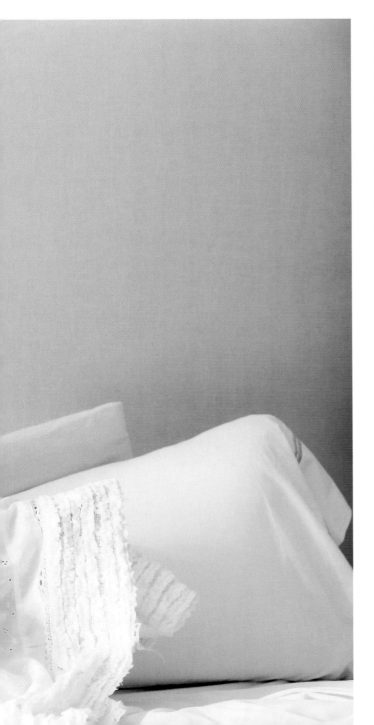

SELMA ON MOTHERHOOD: I never thought I'd cherish every second like I do now. I used to be the kind of person who was like, "When's lunch? When do I get to go to bed? When do I get to go on vacation? When, when, when in the future?" And this child has totally changed me. Now, I can't help but smile and think, "I'm here now."

HARDEST PART: It takes a village, and it's really hard to be the village on your own. But it's still amazingly rewarding.

BEST PART: The way his breath smells like flowers and yogurt—it's the cutest thing.

MOTHERHOOD WISDOM: Let your child be your North Star. If I tried to follow other people's advice, it just wouldn't necessarily fit in with our life and our way of living, and then I'd end up feeling like I'm not doing it right, which just isn't empowering as a mother.

BEST ADVICE: I was so blissed-out when I was pregnant. I had an amazing pregnancy—the hormones felt great, I was really active, I didn't need a lot of sleep, I never had morning sickness after the first month. I was just a totally different person. Then, at my baby shower, a friend of mine said to me, "Oh, no, motherhood is horrible. Prepare." Initially, I was really hurt by that and thought, *I don't want someone in my life who says that kind of negative stuff*. I was kind of shocked. And then, after I gave birth, I just kept going back to her words, and they were actually such a comfort. What she really meant was "Give yourself permission to feel horrible. It's OK to say, 'This isn't bliss yet.'"

PREGNANCY STYLE: When I was pregnant, I never wore black, which was my staple before. It's not that I think black is sad, but I'm just too happy now; it just doesn't feel totally right for me anymore. Instead of buying a lot of maternity clothes, I bought maxi-skirts at Topshop, wore them up above my boobs, and then threw on a belt.

Selma's Uniform

I love dresses, but I'm not totally fit and toned yet. So I wear a lot of long, loose, flowy things. Honestly, it's all about finding cute pajama-like pieces and being able to get out of bed, throw something on, put my head in the sink, and put my hair in a ponytail and still go through the day. I find that as long as I have on a couple of good gold cuffs, a few pieces of jewelry that make me feel like I'm still part of the living, then the rest of my outfit can be a little crumpled.

MAMA STYLE: My style has changed totally since becoming a mom. I used to, and I still do, really love fashion and

really avant-garde pieces—things that definitely had to be dry-cleaned. I don't have any of that in my life right now. Every single thing I wear is breast-accessible, which is not always the chicest. I just call my style "relaxed." I try to find some sweats that still make me happy and aren't obnoxious. If I'm going to be pretty sloppy and casual, I like to do it in a way that I at least think is pretty cute. Trico Field makes great clothing for moms and kids. And then I get to do that really corny thing of matching with my kid, which I've always been a fan of—haters be dammed!

MOTHER-SON MUSINGS: When I wear a dress that has a little bit of sparkle, and I put on some makeup, he'll hold my cheeks and say, "Mama pretty."

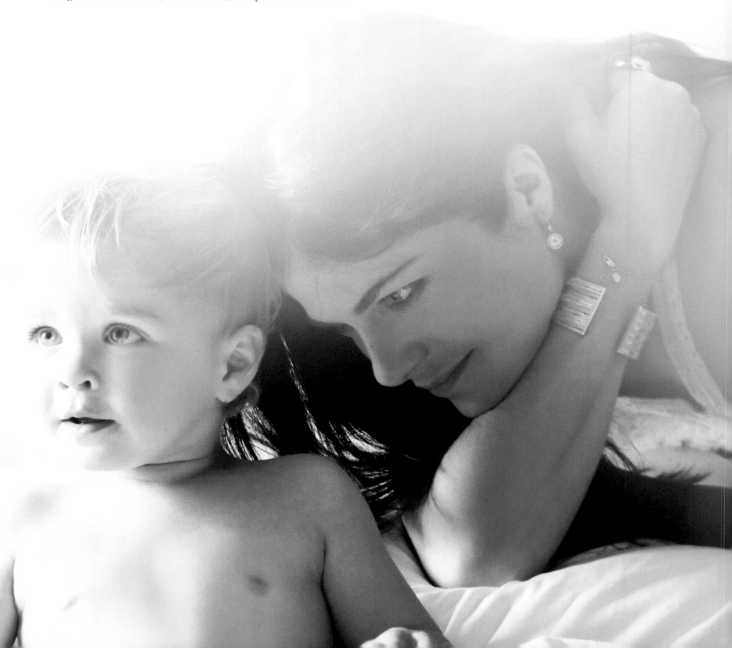

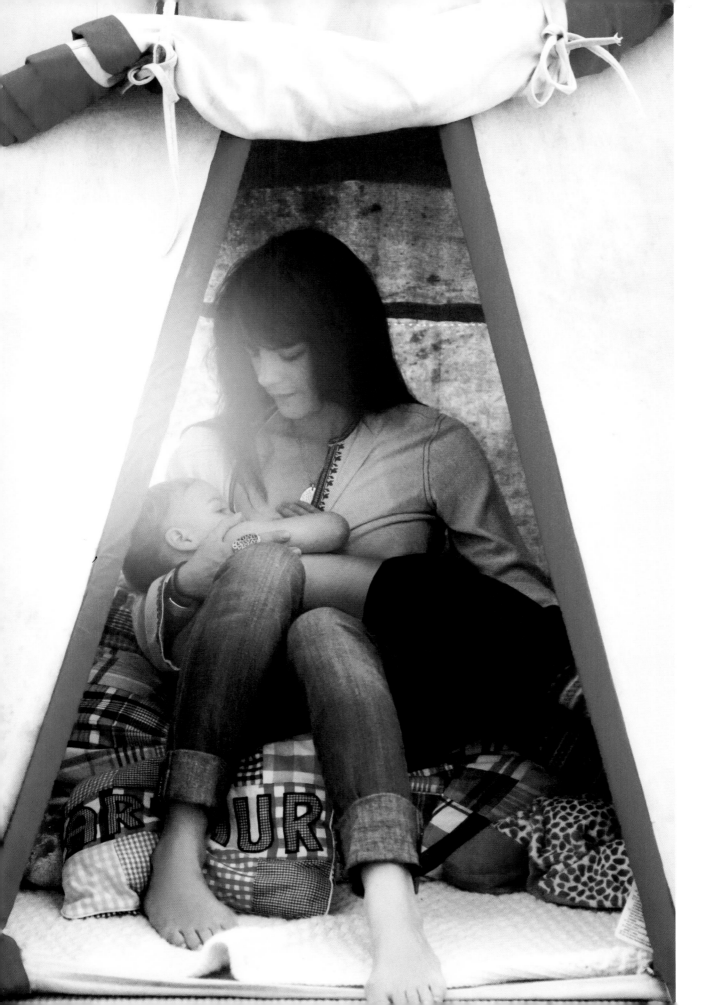

Caroline DEROCHE PASQUIER

GIVENCHY INTERNATIONAL PUBLIC RELATIONS DIRECTOR

———————

Sons Jean and Martin,
photographed at sixteen and eight years old, respectively
Paris, France

Caroline Deroche Pasquier is the definition of Parisian chic. Hands down. She effortlessly mixes vintage YSL and Alaïa with no-name T-shirts and Converse. She can rock a tuxedo like nobody's business and doesn't wear (or need) a stitch of makeup. Oh, and did we mention that her sons are just as chic? (Yes, that is a Givenchy sweatshirt on her sixteen-year-old, seen on page 210.) Her closet has reaped the benefits of an illustrious career working at some of the most iconic French fashion houses—after years at Louis Vuitton, she is now the public relations director for Givenchy. Sons Jean and Martin have clearly inherited her innate sense of style: Her eldest wears vintage almost exclusively, while her eight-year-old has an enviable collection of T-shirts and lives in a vintage varsity jacket from the fifties. With their classically cool wardrobes, Deroche Pasquier and her sons are single-handedly proving that timeless wins out over trendy every time.

CAROLINE ON MOTHERHOOD: A great moment for me was when I realized that these little men we are raising have the right "keys" to live a good life. Our role as parents is to guide them in the best direction, while also accepting who they are. We are here to give them confidence, independence, and respect for themselves. It's not always easy, but it's the most rewarding thing in life!

BEST PART: The love of my boys. They are both so sweet, charming, smart, lovely, and have a good sense of humor. When my younger son says, "Maman, I love you, would you marry me?" I just melt!

HARDEST PART: Fear: It's always there, somewhere inside you.

FAVORITE PART OF THE DAY: I love going out with my older son, just the two of us—sometimes we go to the cinema or to a concert. With Martin, I love the morning when he comes into our bed, right in the middle of us, and cuddles.

WORKING MAMA: I love my work and I need that independence. Then, when I'm home, it's full-on attention and love.

CAROLINE'S STYLE MO: *Quintessential Parisian Chic*
In Caroline Deroche Pasquier's world, Alaïa counts as wardrobe basics, and a heavy-metal spiked Givenchy headband takes the place of perfectly coiffed hair. Instead of makeup, this mom of two adds sparkle to every look with piled-on vintage jewelry, only adding to her irreverent approach to mom style.

PREGNANCY STYLE: Men's shirts and maternity jeans got me through my pregnancy. Other than that, my uniform was a tight dress, long cardigan, flat shoes, and vintage jewelry.

MAMA STYLE: I gravitate toward timeless pieces—like biker jackets, black cashmere, my vintage YSL black tuxedo jacket, and Givenchy T-shirts. I like to pair opposites together: an evening dress paired with natural, undone hair, a silk blouse worn with jeans, or a military jacket and tuxedo pants. And I always buy the same kind of colors—black, navy, dark brown—which makes it much easier to mix and match with the rest of my wardrobe.

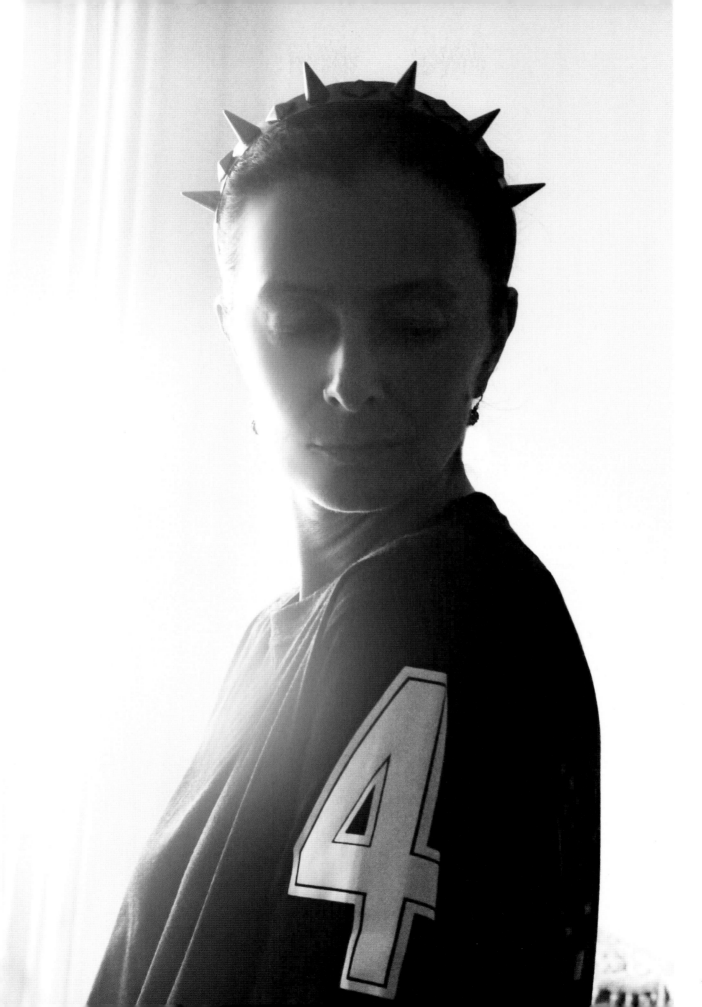

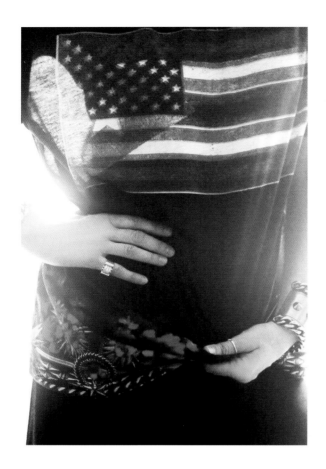

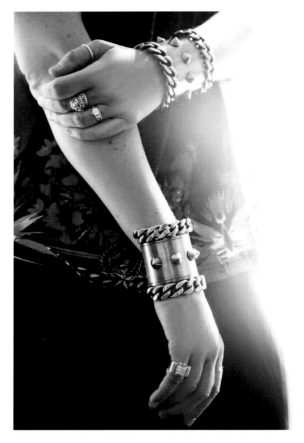

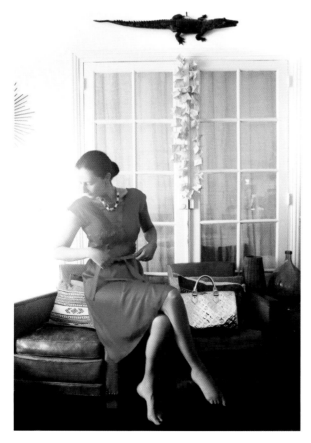

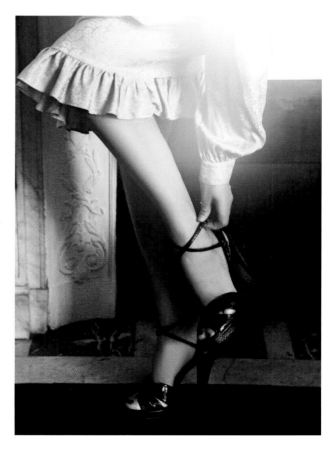

STYLE SENSE

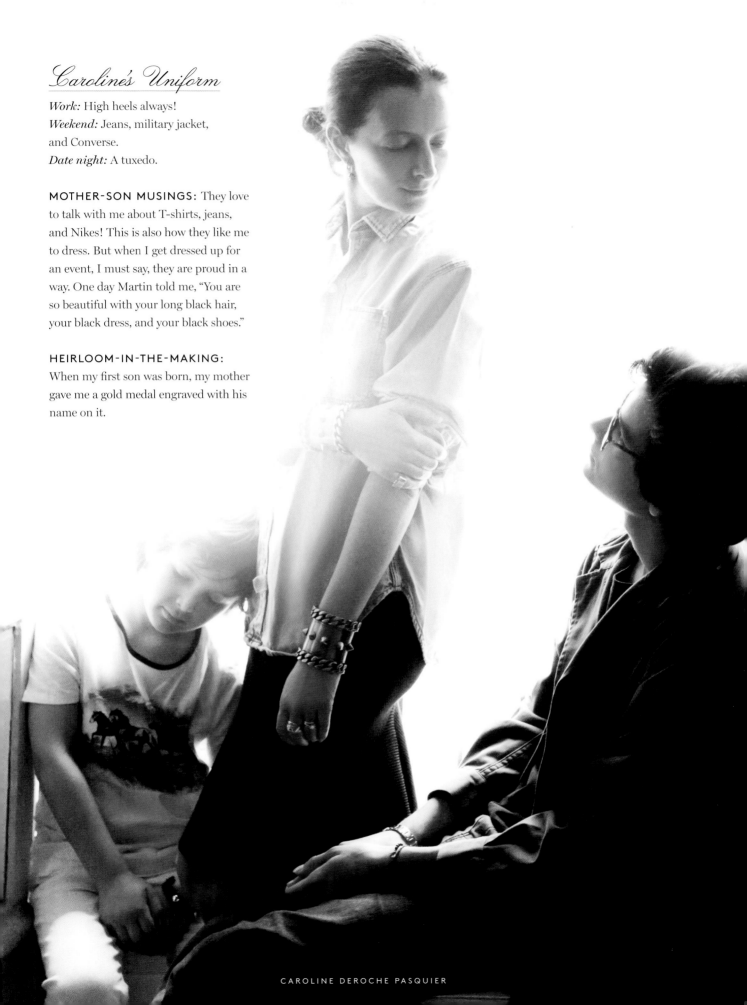

Caroline's Uniform

Work: High heels always!
Weekend: Jeans, military jacket, and Converse.
Date night: A tuxedo.

MOTHER-SON MUSINGS: They love to talk with me about T-shirts, jeans, and Nikes! This is also how they like me to dress. But when I get dressed up for an event, I must say, they are proud in a way. One day Martin told me, "You are so beautiful with your long black hair, your black dress, and your black shoes."

HEIRLOOM-IN-THE-MAKING: When my first son was born, my mother gave me a gold medal engraved with his name on it.

CAROLINE DEROCHE PASQUIER

Jennifer FISHER

JEWELRY DESIGNER

Son Shane and daughter Drew,
photographed at seven and five years old, respectively
New York, New York

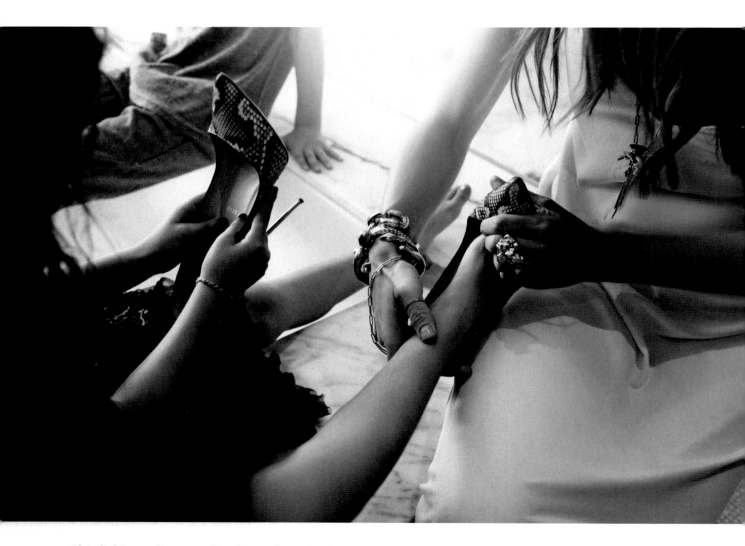

This fashion stylist turned in-demand jewelry designer has most certainly earned her badass spirit. After being diagnosed with cancer at just twenty-seven and undergoing chemotherapy, Fisher went through years of struggling to conceive before getting pregnant naturally and having two healthy children. As a new mom, she was eager to find jewelry she could wear to represent her children while also staying true to her edgy style, so she created her very own letter-stamped necklaces. Friends took notice; soon, orders from major retailers started pouring in, and her now highly coveted jewelry line was born.

JENNIFER ON MOTHERHOOD: I run a tight ship. I've learned that when it comes to discipline, you have to start early.

HARDEST PART: Dealing with the guilt of being a working mom, and the time management involved!

PROUDEST MOMENT: When my son hit his first home run. The look on his face will be forever etched in my mind.

BEST ADVICE: My mother-in-law once told me, "If they are quiet, leave them alone," and it's proven to be so true. People feel the need to overstimulate their kids these days. I like to let them be and imagine and create.

PREGNANCY STYLE: I was obsessed with sticking to regular jeans and wore low-slung, non-pregnancy styles during my entire pregnancy. My saving grace was an elastic waist extender I bought to wear with an amazing, and super-stretchy, pair of Miu Miu jeans. I also bought an army green Chloe cargo jacket (with a chic high collar) two sizes too big and wore it throughout both of my pregnancies until I could barely button it at the end. Overall, I really didn't want to lose myself because I was pregnant. I wanted to adapt to it, embrace it, and accentuate it.

MAMA STYLE: As soon as my son arrived, I immediately stopped wearing my very expensive pieces and opted for cool tees that could be easily washed. I bought some amazing Japanese cargo pants and loose jeans that still had an interesting cut but were comfortable enough to wear while nursing.

Jennifer's Uniform

Work: I leave for work immediately after dropping the kids off, so I am very casual at work and normally have a change of clothes, shoes, and bag to throw on if I'm going out at night straight from the office. That said, I always try to have one piece that is a bit dressier or unexpected. Normally I express myself with jewelry—shocker.
Date night: Leather pants and some vintage rock tees— I keep it simple and comfortable. I feel sexiest in leather pants and high boots. There is something about pants that feels right for me. Almost like a superhero!

MOTHER-DAUGHTER MUSINGS: I encourage Drew to wear whatever she wants. I really want her to have her own sense of style. When I was a kid, my mother would let me walk around in mismatched pants, a tutu, and a weird hat—it was such an amazing feeling. I learned early on that it was OK to express myself and my mood through clothing. In high school, my mother would take me to the fabric store, and I would embellish my vintage finds to make them a bit different—my mother was a huge supporter of my individual style.

Save & Splurge

Save: Tees and tanks—I love H&M layering tanks and T by Alexander Wang tees.
Splurge: Shoes and handbags.

HEIRLOOM-IN-THE-MAKING: As soon as I booked my first huge styling campaign when I was a wardrobe stylist, I bought a classic black, quilted Chanel bag. I'll never forget the amazing feeling of walking out of the store with the bag, which was paid for entirely by my work. I still have it. I'm saving it to give to Drew for one of her birthdays.

MY STYLE IS . . . Utilitarian, unconstrained, and independent.

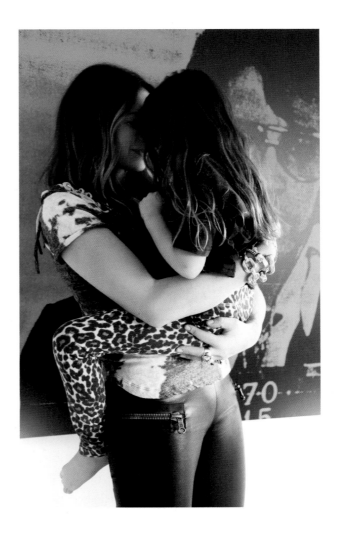

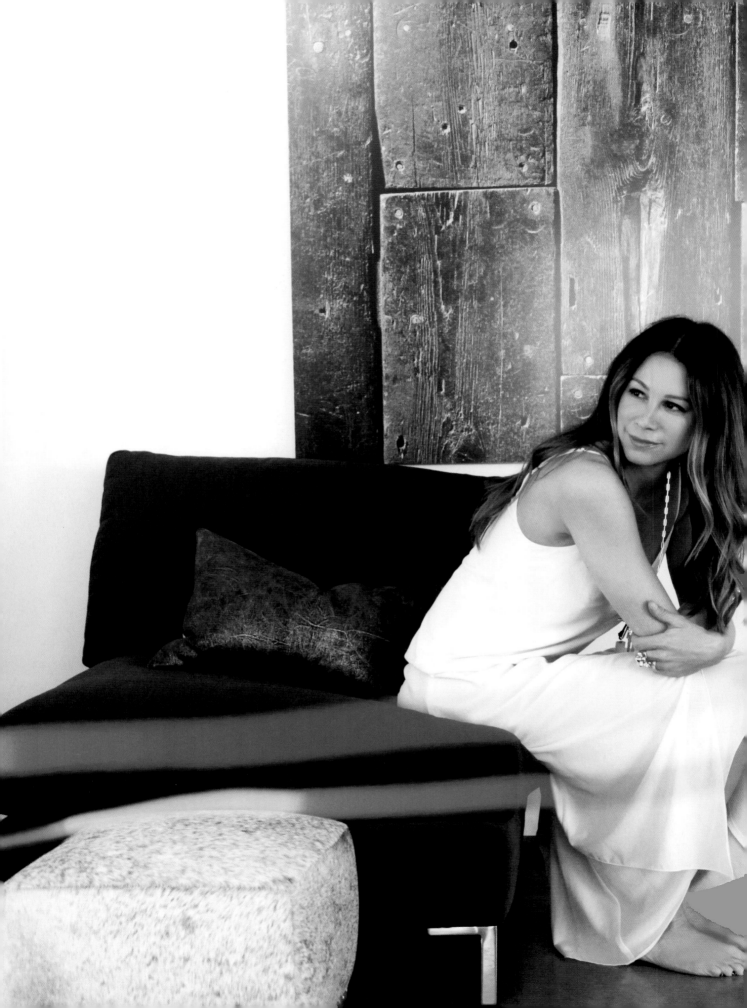

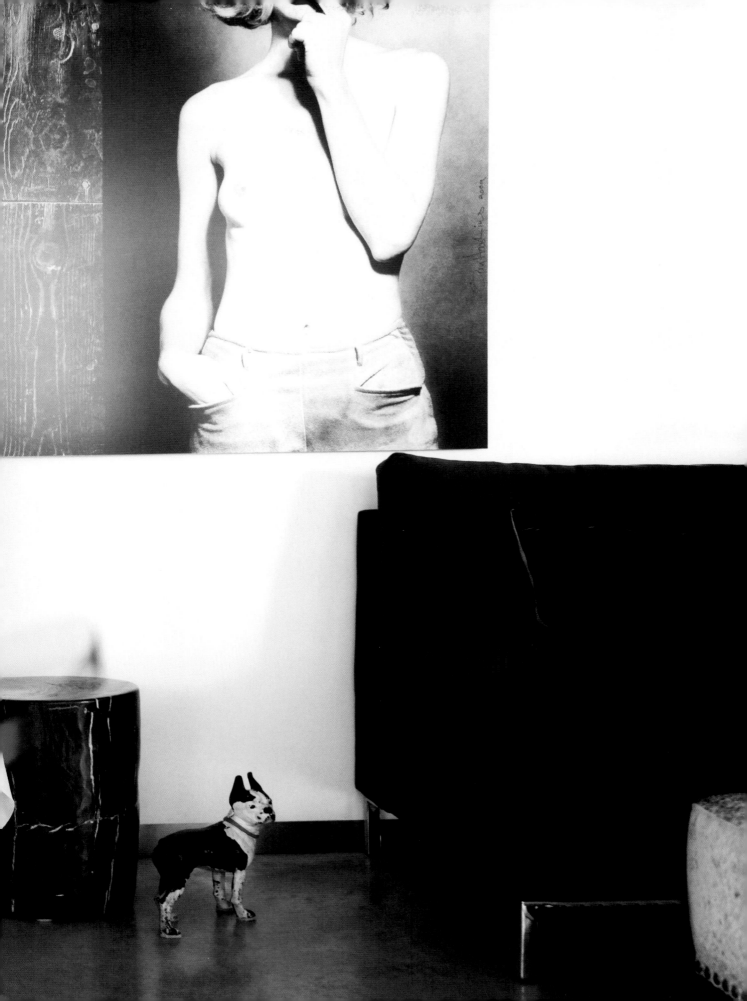

Yasmin SEWELL

FASHION CONSULTANT

Son Knox,
photographed at eighteen months old
London, England

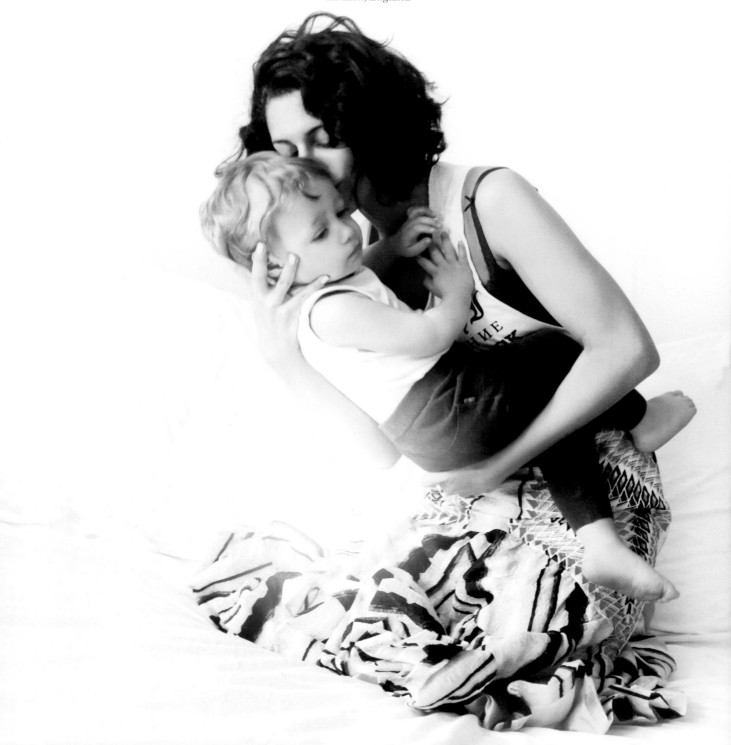

Loved by street-style photographers around the world for her eye-catching, experimental style (not to mention her killer smile), Yasmin Sewell has built a career on tapping into what's cool, way before everyone else catches on. Her foray into fashion began more than a decade ago when the Lebanese beauty moved from Australia to London and, at the age of twenty-two, opened up her own store and started carrying then-unknown brands like Pierre Hardy and A.F. Vandevorst. After a stint as a buyer for influential fashion emporium Browns, Sewell branched out on her own and now runs an in-demand fashion consultancy. As a new mom, her inspiring style has changed only slightly, while her perspective has undergone a drastic shift. Now, she says, "Every day of my life is rewarding, even the tough days."

YASMIN ON MOTHERHOOD: Every moment is fleeting—whether it's a tough phase, a good phase, it will always change. You just can't hold on to any moment for long, so I try to cherish everything.

BIGGEST SURPRISE: I thought I'd have a very strong intuition about what he needed from day one, as I'm a very intuitive person, but I really questioned everything and felt quite unsure for a long time. It took a while for me to get to "Mother knows best."

HARDEST PART: The fear that something could hurt the person you care about so deeply—it makes the bad things in life a lot scarier.

BEST PART: I'm completely in awe of him, and every day he develops as a person. He makes me laugh real, proper laughs and feel proper happiness. The love is out of this world.

FAVORITE PART OF THE DAY: Our dance parties—usually after breakfast and after dinner.

YASMIN'S STYLE MO: *London Cool Girl*
An expert at mixing high and low (case in point: a Peter Pilotto printed skirt paired with a slashed T-shirt), Sewell truly enjoys fashion and never takes herself too seriously. Her wardrobe, is an enviable mix of up-and-coming British designers vintage treasures, and high-end favorites.

PREGNANCY STYLE: During my pregnancy, I limited my wardrobe to just the pieces that still fit, and boxed up the rest. It was nice not to wear a lot of different pieces, and keep my options limited. I wore lots of my husband, Kyle's, oversized shirts with maternity jeans from Topshop. The only other maternity item I bought was bras. For work, I wore dresses from Roksanda Ilincic. It's important to show off your best bits, whether it's your arms, neck, or ankles—keep them out!

MAMA STYLE: I feel sexiest in a good blazer, men's-style jeans, and a high "statement" pump. Since becoming a mom, I have really stayed true to my original style.

Yasmin's Uniform

Work: Man-style jeans, shirts, and blazers
Weekend: Loose dresses and flats, with oversized sweaters
Date night: This is a time to dress up. I wear a lot of young British designers like Peter Pilotto and Mary Katrantzou.

MY STYLE IS . . . Easy, understated, clean.

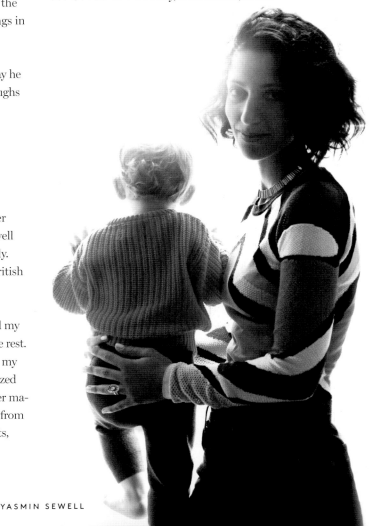

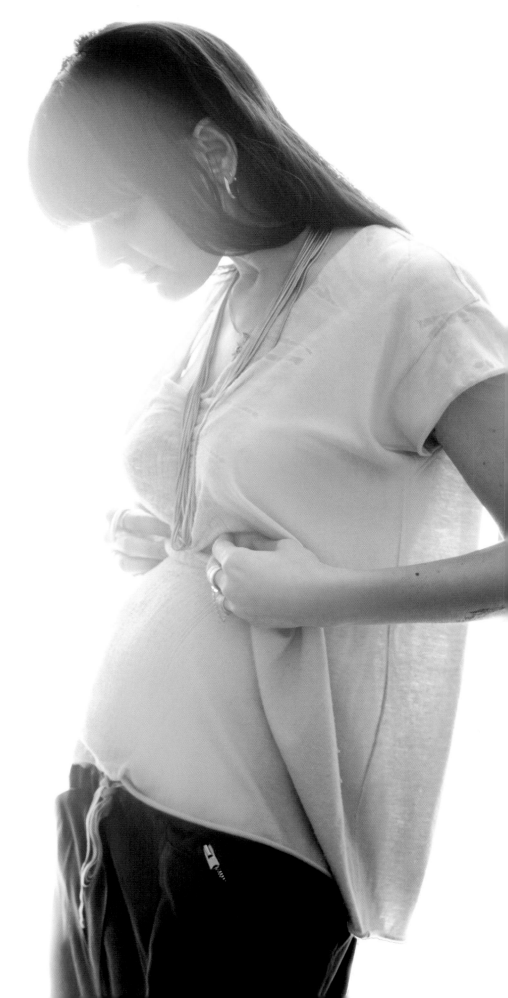

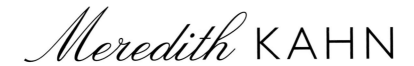

Meredith KAHN

JEWELRY DESIGNER

Daughter Grayson,
photographed at three years old (pictured on page 8)
Brooklyn, New York

Meredith Kahn is the genius behind highly coveted jewelry line, Made Her Think. Her long list of devoted fans flock to her collection for a dose of hard-edged femininity (think double-knuckle rings made of rose gold and diamonds). The designer, four months pregnant in these photos, shows off her growing baby bump and feminine-meets-tough style—from leather leggings to vintage rock tees.

MEREDITH ON MOTHERHOOD: Always do what's in your gut—no one else knows what you or your child needs better than you.

HARDEST PART: It's harder than it looks—it will change you forever.

FAVORITE THINGS: My beautiful and cozy king-size bed (makes me feel like a princess), a home for my keys and Metro card, a comfortable pair of boots, sheepskin slippers, my favorite cozy at-home clothes, and my leather leggings—you don't have to think about what to wear; just pull them on, and you're done.

MEREDITH'S STYLE MO: *Feminine-Meets-Tough*
Don't let the tattoos and leather pants fool you—this Brooklyn mom is a romantic at heart with a touch of rock-star edge. She cleverly mixes flowy, feminine pieces with her spike-, stud-, and chain-adorned jewels for a leather-and-lace look all her own.

PREGNANCY STYLE
Tops: I love Raquel Allegra because her tops allow for a lot of room to grow but sort of form to your body so you look like you still have a shape.
Jeans: Super-low-rise styles with a button fly are the best—just button the bottom ones and use a hairband to thread through the top buttonhole and catch the button. Using this technique, your regular jeans may even get you through

your fifth month, then just size up.
Bras: If you're like me and you jumped numerous bra sizes overnight, you will have to buy new bras. Don't buy the maternity ones yet; you will wear those plenty if you nurse. Find ones with good support and pretty straps that still make you feel sexy.
Leather pants: I took the skinny waistband off my Les Chiffoniers leggings and replaced it with a wider band to make them into maternity pants.

MAMA STYLE: Find a great scarf and wear it so it's handy while you're nursing or even to tie your baby in a sling. When you're a new mom, you're kind of like a nomad when you leave the house. Also, buy a small purse to keep all of your personal items in, and use a cute cotton tote for the baby's needs. Totes work great for men, too.

June AMBROSE

STYLIST

Daughter Summer,
photographed at eight years old
(not pictured: son Chance, ten years old, pictured on page 204)
New York, New York

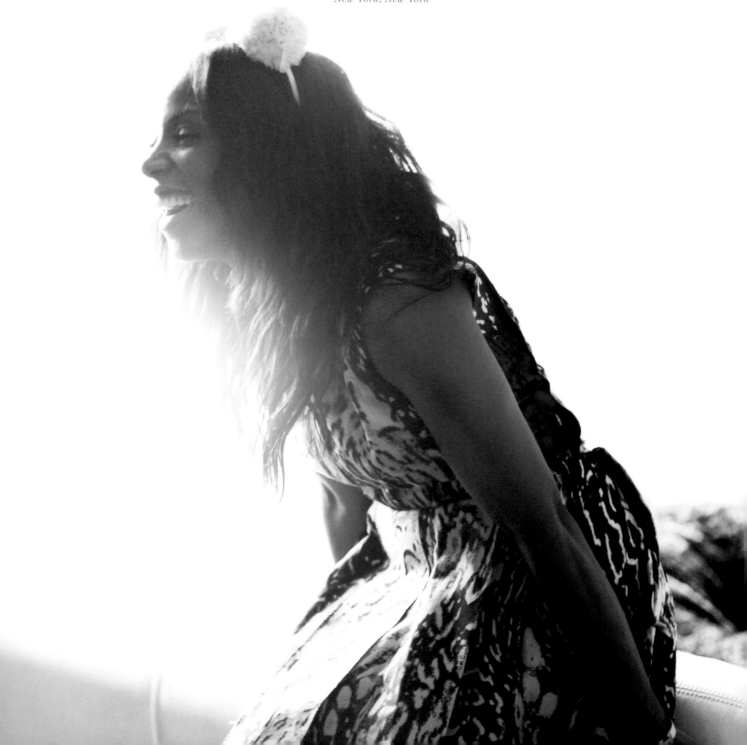

To understand June Ambrose's style, all you need to know is this: Upon the birth of her first child, she commemorated the occasion by buying herself a Birkin bag, which she then used in lieu of a diaper bag. Her style staples—oversize sunglasses, caftans, and Hermès scarves—are a throwback to glamorous icons of the sixties and seventies. While her day job as a stylist and TV personality keeps her plenty busy, it is her cozy home life with her two adorable (and wildly well-mannered) kids that truly grounds her. Through motherhood, Ambrose has "discovered a side of myself I never knew existed."

JUNE ON MOTHERHOOD: Pick your battles. Lead from the back, and let them believe they are in front.

BEST PART: The unconditional love, support, and understanding that my kids offer me—even at an early age. It fuels me like no other.

HARDEST PART: Having to leave them when I don't want to.

WORKING MAMA: I wake up an hour before my kids, and I'm able to get a lot done for myself before having to devote my time to them. Whether it's glam or work, I carve the time out and stick to the schedule.

FAVORITE PART OF THE DAY: The early evening, listening to all their stories. Kids are the best playwrights.

JUNE'S STYLE MO: *Glam Goddess*
With her penchant for six-inch Louboutins, turbans, and Jackie O sunglasses, June Ambrose's style can only be described as fearless. Still, she manages to delicately meld her love of full-on glamour with her more practical, mom-on-the-go side. If her kids had their way, they'd dress her in gowns and leather jackets—"they love when I'm over the top!"

PREGNANCY STYLE: My go-tos were leggings, caftans, oversized Hermès scarves, V-neck tees, and a stretchy waist extension for my jeans. I focused on embracing my new body while staying comfy in empire-waist dresses and tops with an open neckline. I also wore lots of jersey pieces—easy to wear and great for an expanding belly.

JUNE'S UNIFORM: I love drama, so kimonos, big glasses, or leggings paired with an oversize shirt and a fedora hat! I also have several white shirts that I play up and down.

I FEEL MOST SEXY IN . . . Girly, flirty silhouettes and a six-inch pair of heels, of course.

Save & Splurge

Save: Trendy fashion.
Splurge: Jewelry—I know my daughter will appreciate it later in life.

MOTHER-CHILD MUSINGS: I tell my daughter that she's beautiful on the inside first, and the outside shows off your spirit!

MY STYLE IS . . . Fearless, sassy, and metropolitan.

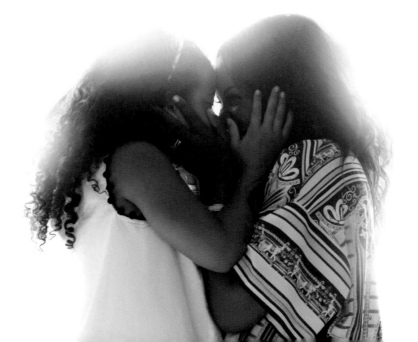

Sara BLAKELY

SPANX FOUNDER

Son Lazer,
photographed at three years old
New York, New York

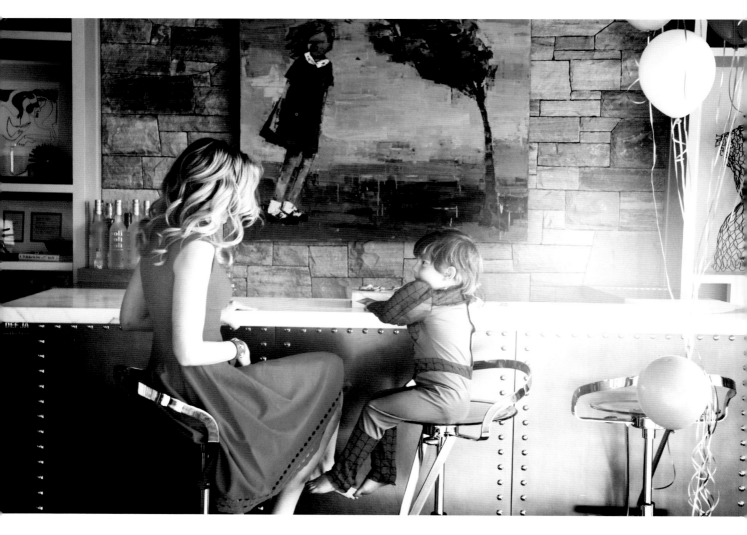

Before the age of thirty, Sara Blakely had already revolutionized the way women dress. Spanx, her billion-dollar company, accomplished the impossible: Suddenly, shapewear was considered cool. Three years ago, Blakely's life was once again turned upside down when she welcomed her first child into the world. While she admits that her body has changed, her approach to style hasn't. She gravitates toward color and whimsical prints—her son, on the other hand, is all about comfort: "I try to get him to wear 'cool' jeans, but he says, 'Mommy, I don't want to look cool. I want to be comfortable!'

SARA ON MOTHERHOOD: When I was growing up, my father used to encourage my brother and me to fail. This changed the course of my life. When a parent gives you permission to fail, and even celebrates it, life opens up to you in amazing ways. You take more risks and view failure as not trying instead of the outcome. My son is only three, but I will be encouraging him to fail, spread his wings, and maybe even high-five him too when he tells me he tried out for something and was horrible at it!

HARDEST PART: Breast-feeding! Everyone focuses on the birth, but breast-feeding was by far one of the hardest things I've ever done in my life. I didn't sleep through the night for seven months.

BEST PART: The arms-thrown-around-your-neck, heart-pressed-against-heart hugs!

WORKING MAMA: My motto is "Think, prioritize, delegate what you can, and let it go . . ." I've found that I'm more effective when I compartmentalize my day—I have a mom section and a work section to each day. As a result, I'm more present and less scattered.

PROUDEST MOMENT: Giving more than twenty million dollars away to help women. I just can't believe that the girl who failed the LSAT and sold fax machines door-to-door for years has been able to give back in such a big way.

FAVORITE PART OF THE DAY: Bedtime. I get into bed with Lazer and read him books. I scratch his back until he falls asleep.

SARA'S STYLE MO: *Playfully Chic*
As a mom and a CEO, Sara Blakely's number-one priority when getting dressed is function. So instead of heels, she can most often be found in chic flats or Converse. With her playful use of prints, color, and texture, it's no wonder she describes her personal style as "spontaneous, comfortable, and eclectic."

PREGNANCY STYLE: I didn't adjust my style that much—I just bought bigger sizes in regular clothes. I did, however, live in maternity jeans and my Spanx Power Mama® (our maternity shaping short). As my boobs grew, our bra, Spanx Bra-llelujah!®, grew with me because of the all-hosiery back. I also used the bra during breast-feeding, as it was easy to lift up.

Sara's Uniform

School run: I spend half the day in my Spanx Active workout pants, a T-shirt, and jeans. I call it the extended workout look—it's so easy! So that's what I usually wear when I drop my son off at school.
Work: It's usually jeans and a cute top.
Date nights: Jeans and an even cuter top! Did I mention I like jeans?!

MAMA STYLE: I have been to many events all glammed-out, only to look down and realize I have severely chipped nail polish. Not subtle chips, but half the polish gone from my nails, and some nails with no polish left on them at all. I've been that way my whole life. My grandmother still chases me around with nail polish remover. I like to wear fun fake jewelry from gumball machines, and even wore an edible candy jewelry necklace with my gown to the SAG Awards. My style secret is maintaining a sense of humor; polished I am not!

I FEEL SEXIEST IN . . . Jeans and anything that makes me look good but is still comfortable. I don't subscribe to the saying "beauty is pain." I call that B.S. (Before Spanx). Basically, once women got involved, we proved that things can be a lot more comfortable—that's what Spanx did for the girdle.

MOTHER-SON MUSINGS: The other day, I put on a floral dress to give a speech, and he stopped in the hall and said, "Wow, Mommy, you look so beautiful." So he either loves floral dresses or was just so surprised to see me in something other than jeans.

Save & Splurge

Save: I have a lucky red backpack I carried for years instead of a purse. So I've saved lots of money on purses through the years. I carry the same one forever. Now my red backpack is hanging in a glass case at Spanx.
Splurge: I splurge on experiences for friends and family, things that save me time, organic food, and water in glass bottles.

MY STYLE IS . . . Spontaneous, comfortable, eclectic.

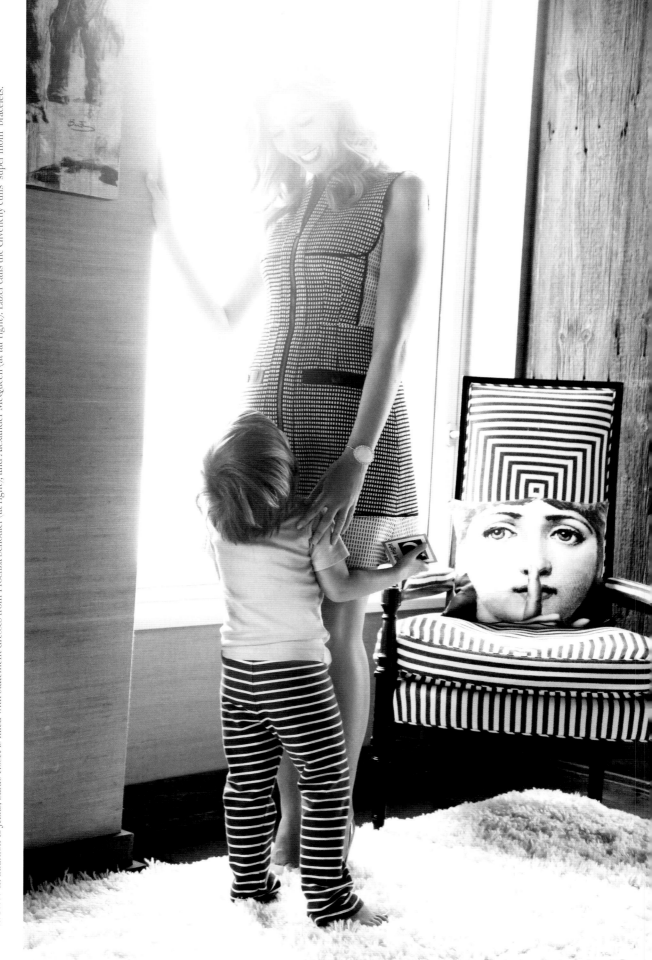

RIGHT: In addition to jeans, Sara's closet is filled with statement dresses from Proenza Schouler (at right), and Alexander McQueen (at far right). Lazer calls the Givenchy cuffs "super mom" bracelets.

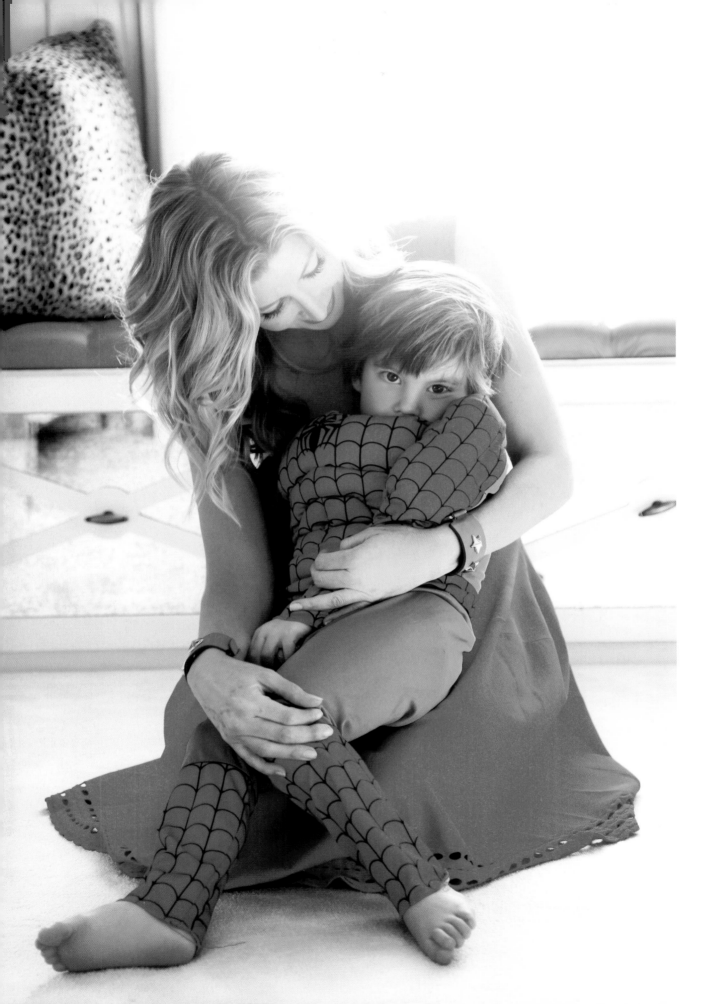

"I like to try everything. I think fashion should be free and experimental . . . Tuesday always wants me to wear high heels and is disappointed if I lack accessories."

—MINNIE MORTIMER, *fashion designer*

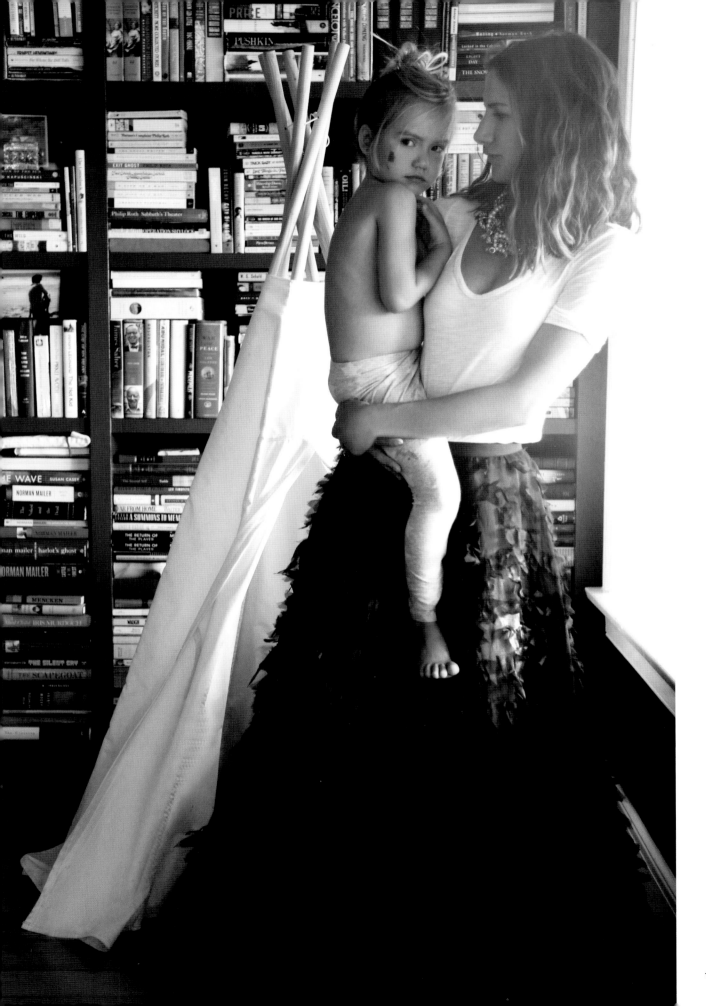

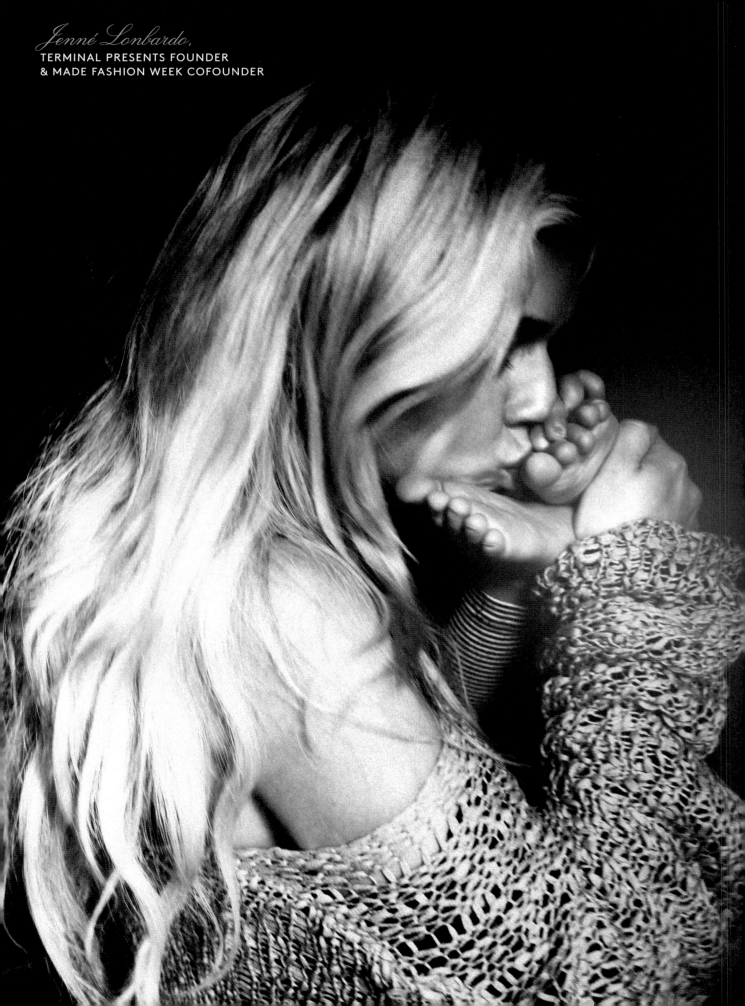

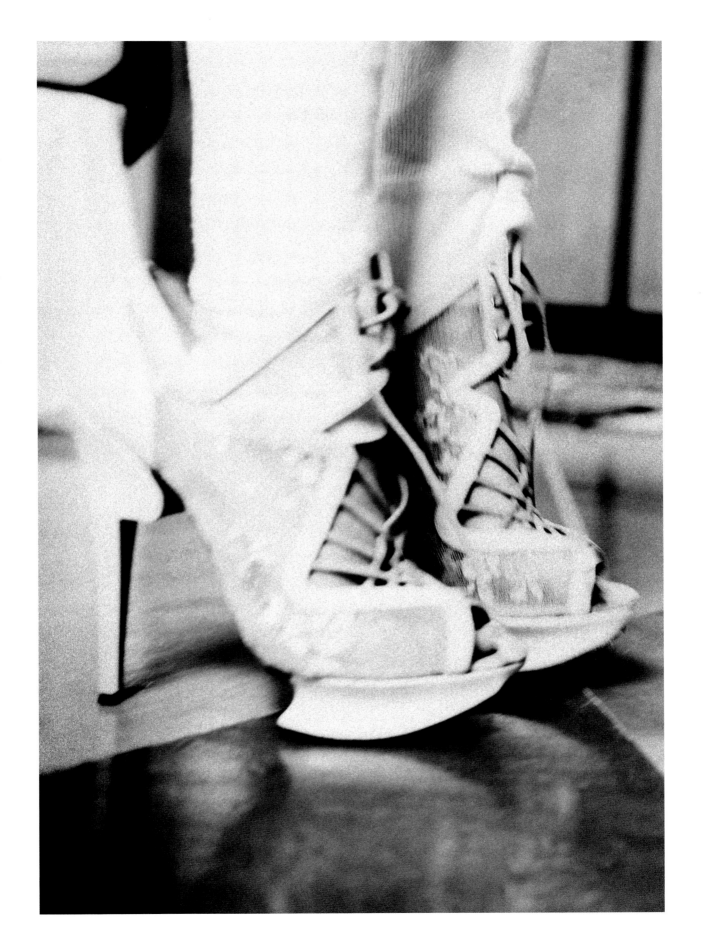

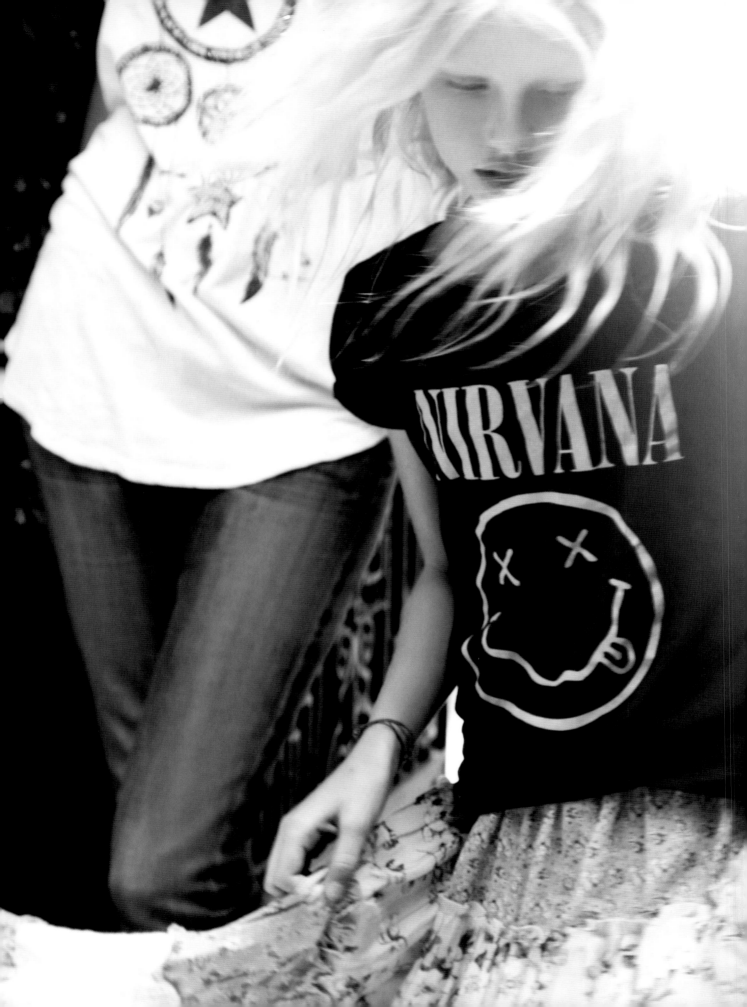

CHAPTER EIGHT

Style Sense ... for Kids

JESSIE RANDALL, *Loeffler Randall founder* · REBECCA TAYLOR, *fashion designer*

WHITNEY BROMBERG HAWKINGS, *Tom Ford international SVP of communications*

CLARE VIVIER, *accessories designer* · JEANNE YANG, *stylist & designer*

*D*espite having a healthy appetite for fashion and accessories, most of the moms we feature on The Glow readily admit that in the beginning, at least, they would rather spend money on clothes for their babies than for themselves. Even before the baby arrives, the strong desire to collect scrumptious and stylish pieces to wrap your child in one day is part of the process of preparing. For me, the idea of becoming a mom became that much more real when my husband brought home a handful of striped cotton onesies from Paris. Holding those teensy pieces in my hands helped me to visualize what it would be like to hold my child. With the irresistibly adorable array of options out there, shopping for babies' and kids' clothes is better than ever.

Brooklyn mom of three, and Loeffler Randall founder, Jessie Randall admits that she tried, for as long as possible, to dress her kids like "little French boys." As her sons have gotten older, Randall has put away the Peter Pan–collar shirts (for now) and leans more toward well-cut pieces with an interesting design element. Three of the style-setting moms featured in this chapter—Randall, Rebecca Taylor, and Tom Ford International SVP of Communications Whitney Bromberg Hawkings, all moms to sons—are single-handedly proving that boys' clothes, notorious for being too blah and brown, have become infinitely more exciting in recent years. The trick to styling the under-ten set—boy or girl—is simple; just stick to the three C's: comfort, cut, and a little something cool. Of course, there's also the fourth C: cost. One trick each mom can agree on is that buying up in size allows them to spend a little more on quality without losing money in the long run.

Here, we explore the brands, styling tips, and go-to pieces cherished by these fashionable women known for their own enviable style. They show us how to translate their favorite design elements—from rock-and-roll tees and bright colors to vintage treasures and French-inspired stripes—into their child's wardrobe. If all else fails, keep this piece of advice in mind from model-turned-mom Kirsty Hume: "I let my daughter put things together on her own—it's amazing what she comes up with!"

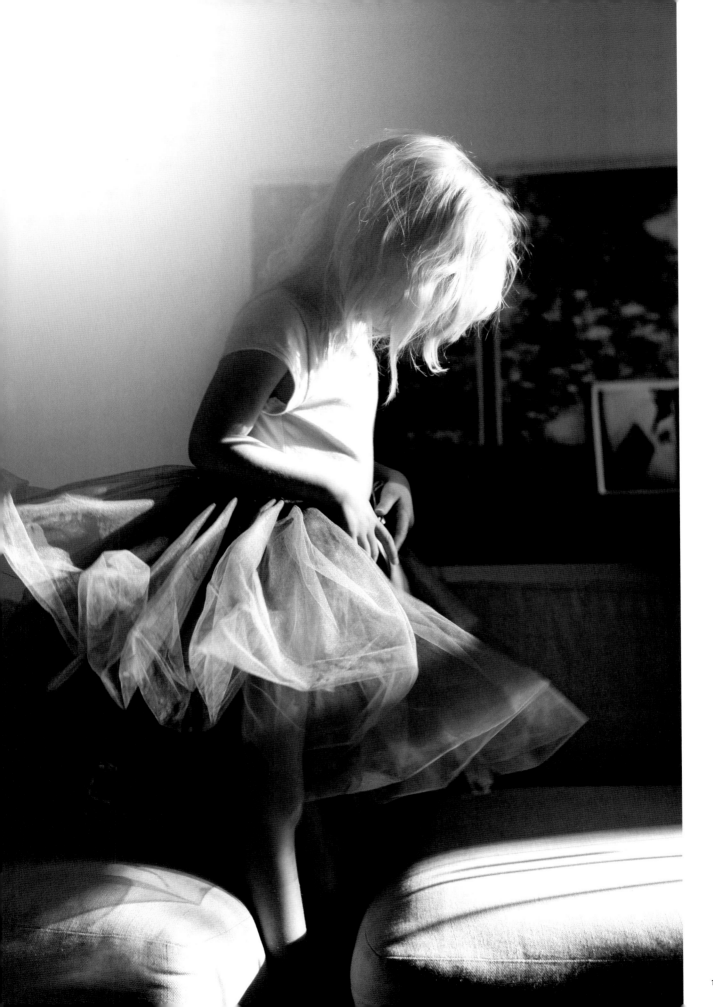

Jessie RANDALL

FOUNDER OF LOEFFLER RANDALL

Twins Casper and Liam and son Harry,
photographed at six and two and a half years old, respectively
Brooklyn, New York

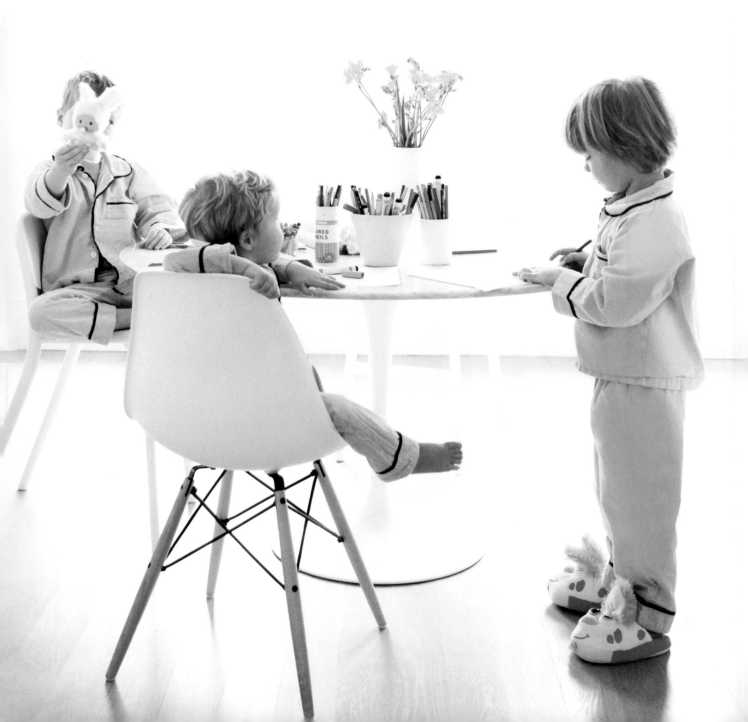

Loeffler Randall, known for creating cool-girl accessories with just a hint of irreverence, has established itself as the go-to brand for unique, wearable pieces. Its founder, Jessie Randall, lives and breathes the brand's offbeat charm in both her personal style and enviable home décor. Randall's Brooklyn town house has a serene feel, with creamy walls and neutral furnishings. When it comes to dressing her three boys, she's all about creating a preppy-cool vibe—think pastels mixed with brights. Lucky for her, sons Casper, Liam, and Harry will wear "pretty much whatever I lay out for them, as long as it is comfortable."

JESSIE ON MOTHERHOOD: It's important for me to take time for myself. I want my boys to see me taking care of myself, not only taking care of others.

HARDEST PART: At work, I sometimes feel like I am shortchanging my kids. At home, it's tough to give them each the individual time they deserve.

BEST PART: Having the sweetest, kindest, most loving boys who just shower me with love and kisses.

FAVORITE PART OF THE DAY: I love our downtime on the weekends, working on an art project or making holiday decorations together.

MY BOYS' STYLE IS . . . A little preppy, but cool. Casper's surfer-style haircut is modeled on the little boy in *Kramer vs. Kramer*.

FAVORITE STYLES: I love to see my boys in pastel colors and bright blues. As long as I could possibly get away with it, I dressed them like little French boys—in sweet brands like Makie, Flora and Henri, and Olive Juice. As the boys have gotten older, they've started to wear a lot of Crewcuts.

Go-To Pieces

* Crewcuts shirts, sweatshirts, and sweatpants
* Clarks shoes
* Patagonia jackets
* Villebrequin bathing suits
* Salt Water sandals for dressing up in the summertime and on vacation
* I also love a Peter Pan–collar shirt, so I always keep one around.

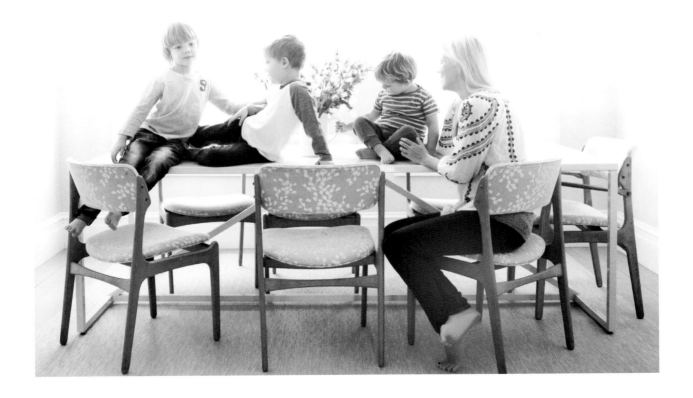

Whitney BROMBERG HAWKINGS

TOM FORD INTERNATIONAL SVP OF COMMUNICATIONS

Sons Baron and Snowden,
photographed at five and two years old, respectively
London, England

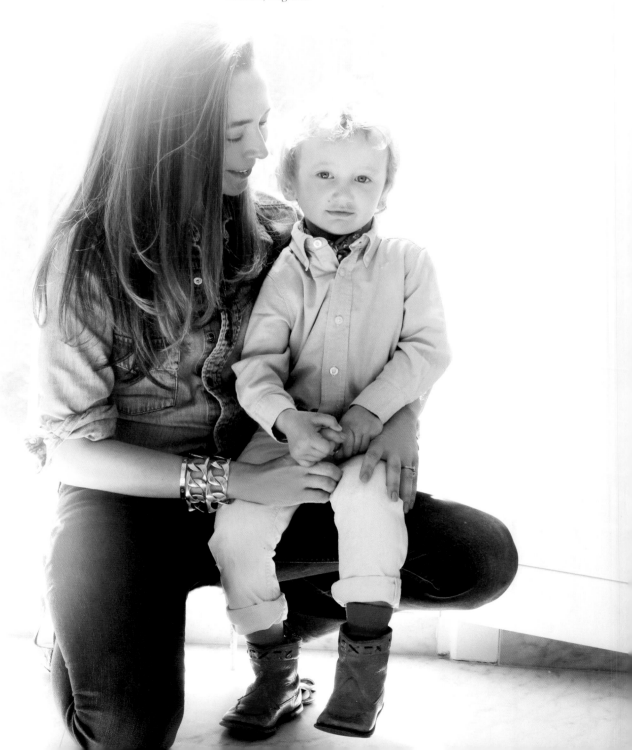

Whitney Bromberg Hawkings began her career in fashion as Tom Ford's devoted assistant. Fifteen years later, the mother of two is now the senior vice president of communications for Europe, the Middle East, India, and Australia. With her infectious energy and impeccable taste, she manages to make it all look so easy. Her secret, she admits, is a wonderful husband and a great nanny. While the balance is a constant struggle, and she wishes she could pick her boys up from school every day, their precious mornings together keep her going throughout the day.

WHITNEY ON MOTHERHOOD: The key is to prioritize and make sure that my children always come first in things that matter. For me, those things are bath time and bedtime. No matter how busy I am, I am always home in time to give my kids a bath and put them to sleep.

HARDEST PART: Patience.

BEST PART: Every single little thing.

FAVORITE PART OF THE DAY: When they come bounding into our bed in the morning for a cuddle. Their sleep-tousled hair and delicious little morning breath is my definition of heaven.

MY BOYS' STYLE IS . . . Vintage and unexpected.

FAVORITE STYLES: I love them in vintage denim, with bandanas in bright colors tied around their necks like little scarves. While I do love seeing the boys in bright colors, I also think you can't go wrong with navy accessorized by little bits of red. We are lucky that the boys have always loved the attention they receive when they are dressed nicely, so they are always asking to get dressed up and have a spray of Tom Ford's Neroli Portofino on the collar of their shirts!

Go-To Pieces

★ Bonpoint for jeans in different colors
★ Crewcuts for cashmere sweaters and shirts, all thrown in with a bit of vintage to keep it from being too expected
★ Vintage Levi's jackets and Wrangler denim vests

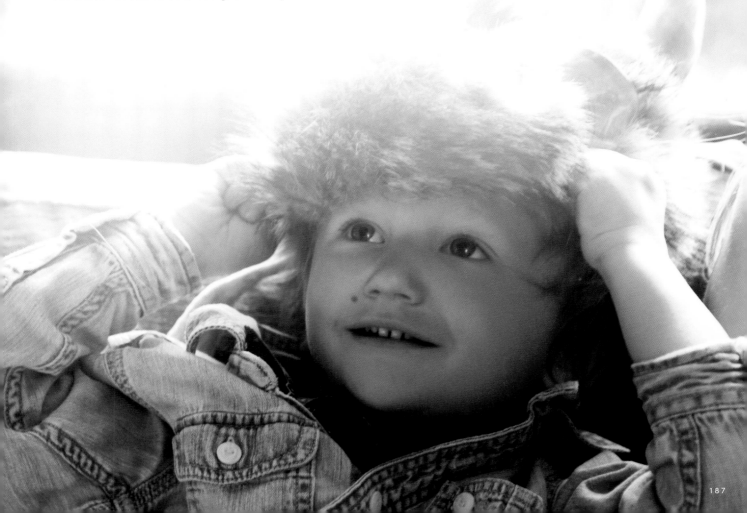

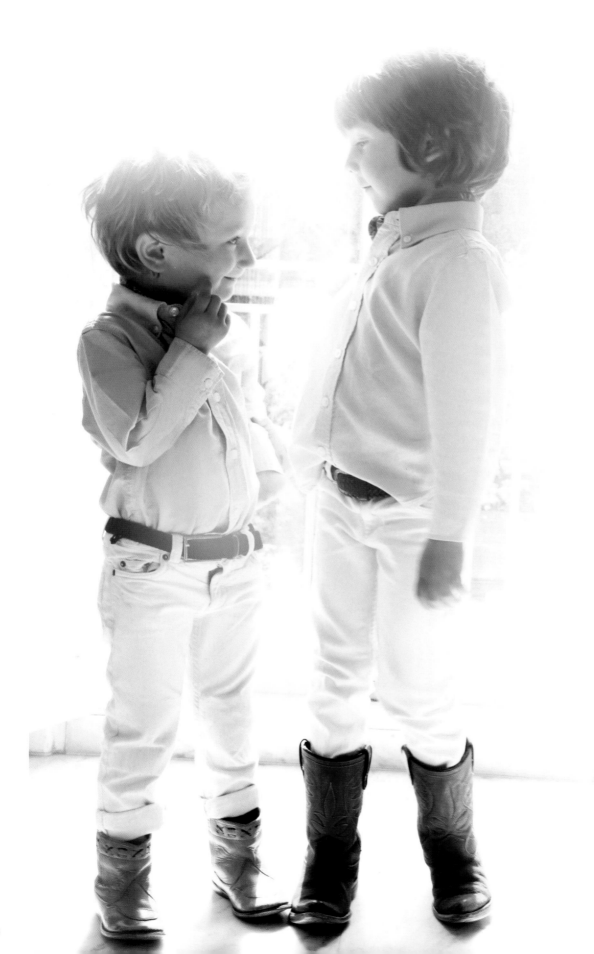

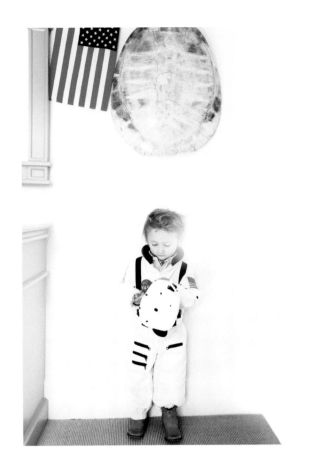

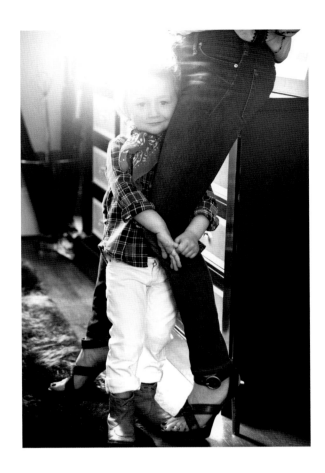

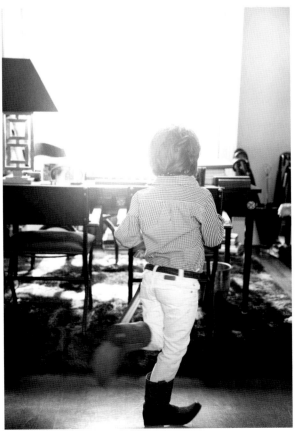

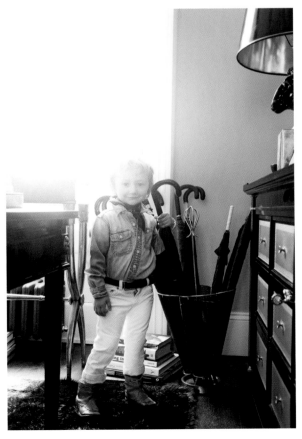

Rebecca TAYLOR

FASHION DESIGNER

———————————

Twins Zoe and Isabel and son Charlie,
photographed at six and four years old, respectively
Brooklyn, New York

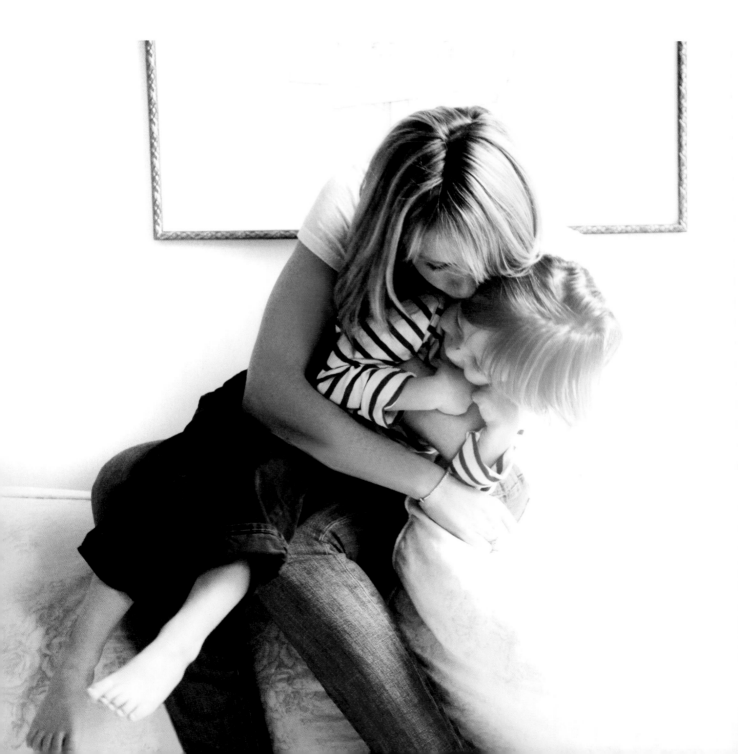

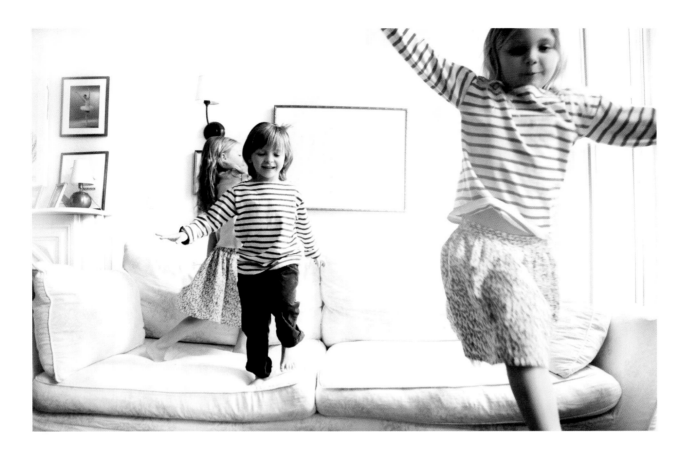

Rebecca Taylor's Brooklyn brownstone embodies some of the same sensibilities that have made women around the world fall in love with her eponymous clothing line: timeless, feminine, and vintage inspired. With three young children running around, the home feels at once lived-in and chic (not an easy combination to pull off). When it comes to her own style, and the pieces she picks out for her son and twin daughters, Taylor is all about simplicity: Striped shirts serve as the centerpiece of all of their wardrobes. And the busy mom admits, she and the kids often end up wearing the same outfit. Clearly, good style runs in the family.

REBECCA ON MOTHERHOOD: I try to be in the moment as much as I can when I'm with the kids. At night, I lie down, respond to them, and just chat about what's on their mind.

HARDEST PART: How relentless it is—every morning you wake, and there they are! Also, every time you turn around they are hungry again!

BIGGEST SURPRISE: When I realized that children are who they are from birth. I always thought I would have more influence on how their personalities would shape up.

BEST PART: Everything! I was destined to be a mom. My children are my lifeblood now. I race home after work to snuggle and hang out.

PROUDEST WORK MOMENT: The Duchess of Cambridge wearing one of my designs.

FAVORITE GIRLS' STYLES: I love dressing my girls. I'm not really a pink kind of girl myself, so I don't really go in that direction for them. I gravitate toward lots of Liberty prints and clean cashmere. Striped tees and gray leggings are a must.

FAVORITE BOYS' STYLES: Charlie has a real uniform: striped tee, gray sweatpants, Converse, and Spiderman knickers!

MOTHER-SON STYLE: Surprisingly, I end up wearing matching outfits with my son, not the girls! Not on purpose; we just like the same things.

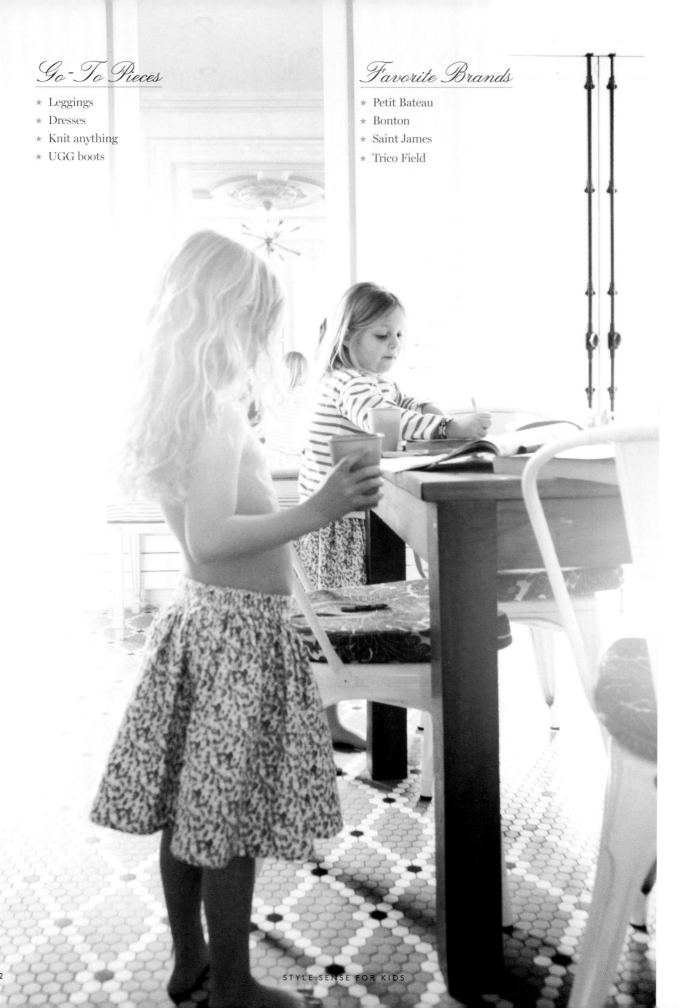

Go-To Pieces

* ★ Leggings
* ★ Dresses
* ★ Knit anything
* ★ UGG boots

Favorite Brands

* ★ Petit Bateau
* ★ Bonton
* ★ Saint James
* ★ Trico Field

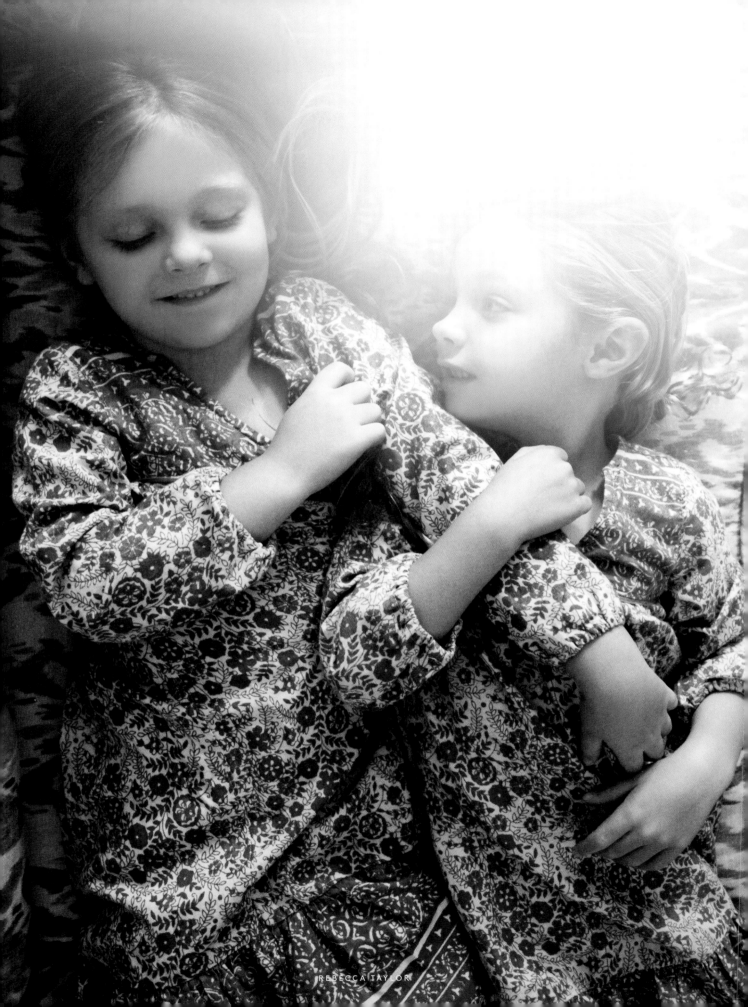

REBECCA TAYLOR

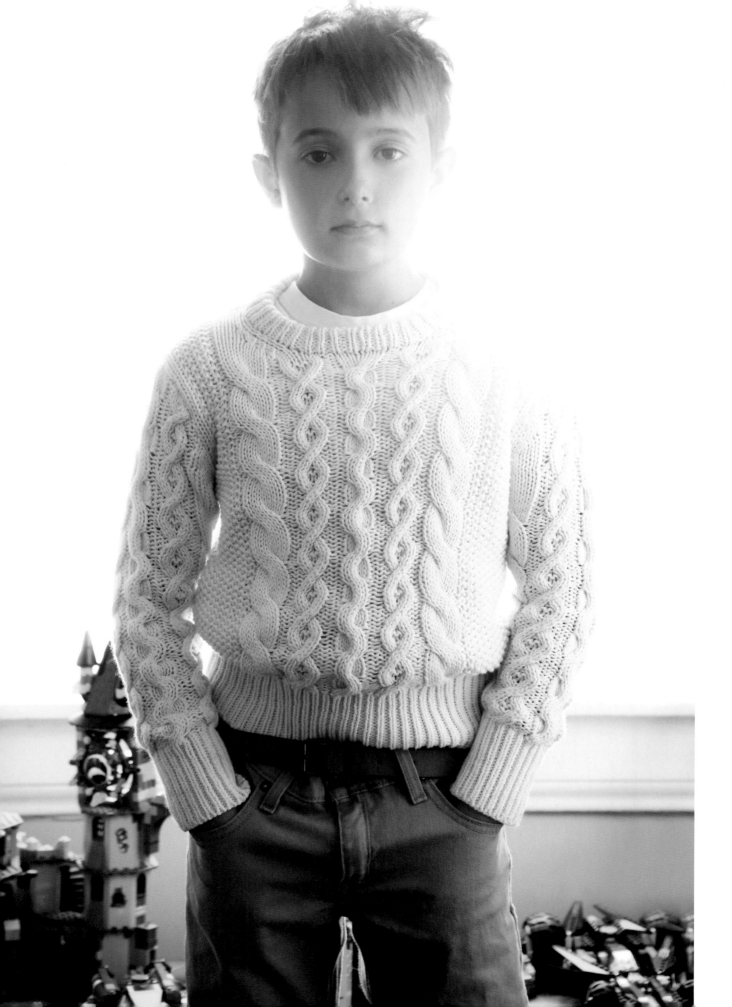

Clare VIVIER

Son Oscar,
photographed at nine years old
Los Angeles, California

Clare Vivier's namesake line of minimal-chic handbags has gained a fiercely devoted following thanks to her desire to stay true to what women really want. At the end of the day, Vivier realizes that quality, versatility, and a touch of je ne sais quoi get the job done. Her irreverent approach extends beyond bags to her home décor, personal style, and even her son's unexpected fashion choices. The bilingual ten-year-old (Vivier met her Parisian husband while living abroad) has a penchant for pairing slightly cropped khakis with classic white T-shirts and chunky, shrunken sweaters. The result: a look that's unique and playful while still delivering on comfort. While Vivier admits that she's heavily influenced her son's cool look, she also realizes "he has a strong sense of style, and little flourishes of his own." Clearly, she's taught him well.

CLARE ON MOTHERHOOD: I am so proud of him for working hard at school and really caring about doing well. He is self-assured, and that is very satisfying for a parent.

HARDEST PART: I wish I was better at planning meals, organizing toys, and just organizing all of his stuff in general.

BEST LESSONS: Being polite, opening doors for women, and letting them go first! It sounds outdated, but I think it's a good lesson to think of others before yourself—why not start with women?

FAVORITE STYLES: I definitely shy away from super boy-centric styles and instead like to see him in plain white T-shirts and slim-fitting pants. I think children are so beautiful and should just dress simply, or else it takes away from their beauty.

MOTHER-SON STYLE: He generally doesn't comment on what I'm wearing, except for when he called a pair of my beloved Isabel Marant striped pants "circus pants."

SHOPPING TIPS: I stock up on classic white T-shirts from Hanes and Fruit of the Loom—they're the best!

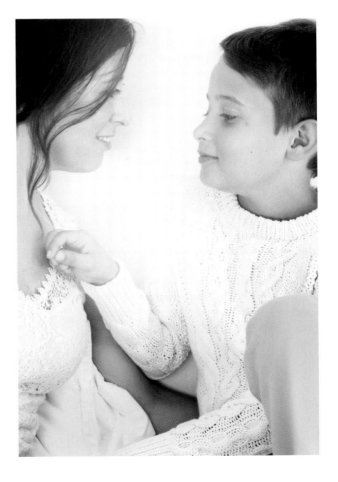

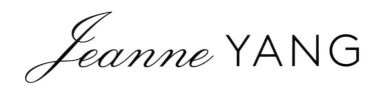

Jeanne YANG

STYLIST & DESIGNER

Twin daughters Zoey and Sydney,
photographed at nine years old
Los Angeles, California

As one half of the fashion label Holmes & Yang, Jeanne Yang has a knack for creating successful duos. Case in point: daughters Zoey and Sydney. Old souls at heart, the identical twins finish each other's sentences and, as their mom puts it, are built-in best friends. When she's not soaking up family time in her glass-enclosed, Richard Neutra–designed tree house, Yang is traveling the world styling clients like Brad Pitt and Christian Bale. In 2008, after noticing a gap in the fashion market, Yang and longtime client (and friend) Katie Holmes decided to create a high-end line for working moms just like themselves—a uniform of sorts to simplify women's lives. Two careers, two kids, a dog, and a lizard named Dragon—it's all in a day's work for this energetic powerhouse.

JEANNE ON MOTHERHOOD: The best moment of my life was when my ladies were born, and it's only gotten better.

HARDEST PART: Getting out of the car at the airport to leave on a trip, with both of them crying and saying to hurry back.

BEST PART: Coming back from trips and being greeted with a flood of kisses and love notes—I feel like I have presents waiting for me when I walk in the door.

BEST ADVICE: Speak to your children as you would like to be spoken to.

FAVORITE STYLES: I love to see my girls in bright colors, especially reds and pinks. I also love the way they mix patterns, polka dots, and plaids. My favorite addition to each outfit is the way they always add belts to every look. It's not necessarily the clothes but the way kids put pieces together that's the most interesting.

GO-TO PIECES: Zoey has an old Ralph Lauren cashmere sweater she has worn since she was three—it is so cute as the sleeves are now three-quarter and it looks very Audrey Hepburn. Because it is made so well, it still looks great.

Sydney's favorite piece is a T-shirt with a Chihuahua with glasses on it from Crewcuts. She wears it twice a week, so we bought a second one in a larger size—I don't know what she will do when it starts to fall apart.

SHOPPING TIPS: Vintage clothing is not only economical, but it's also better made most of the time and, of course, one-of-a-kind. I love finding vintage pieces and altering things down to the girls' sizes. I also tend to buy quality, better-made designer pieces. My girls have had floor-length dresses for years which they still wear, even though they only reach their knees now. These dresses are classic cuts, well made, and have stood up to the wear and tear of many years and fleeting fashion trends.

STYLE EVOLUTION: The girls have finally started to wear pants, due in part to their newfound interest in skateboarding. I have been trying for almost ten years to get my ladies to try pants or jeans, and they have only now started to add them to their wardrobe. Skirts and dresses composed every outfit, even their school uniforms. I can't wait to see how they will style their pant looks.

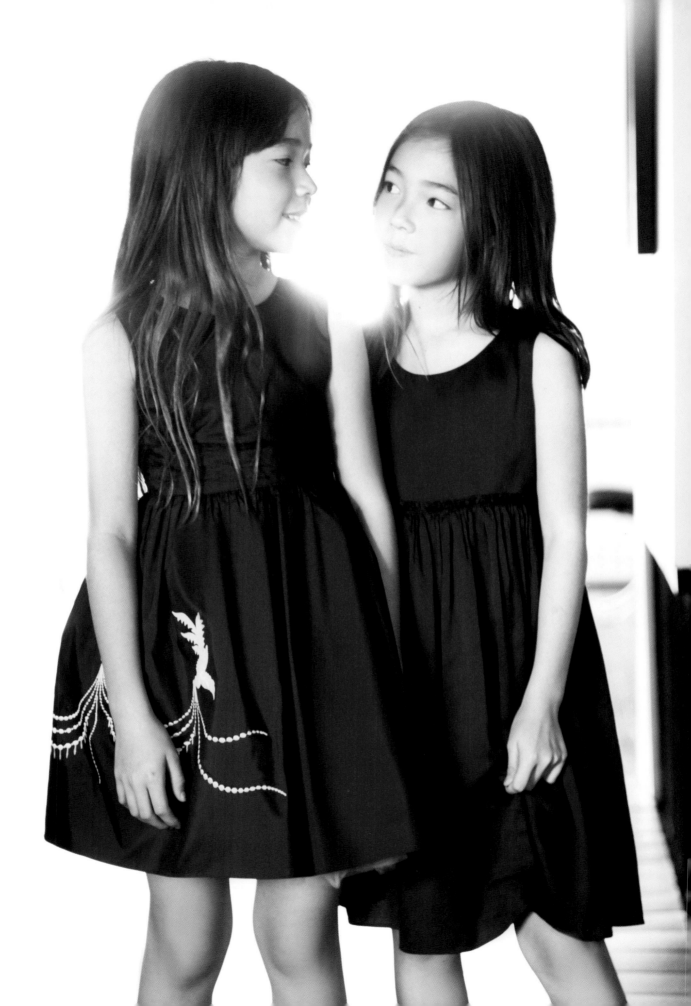

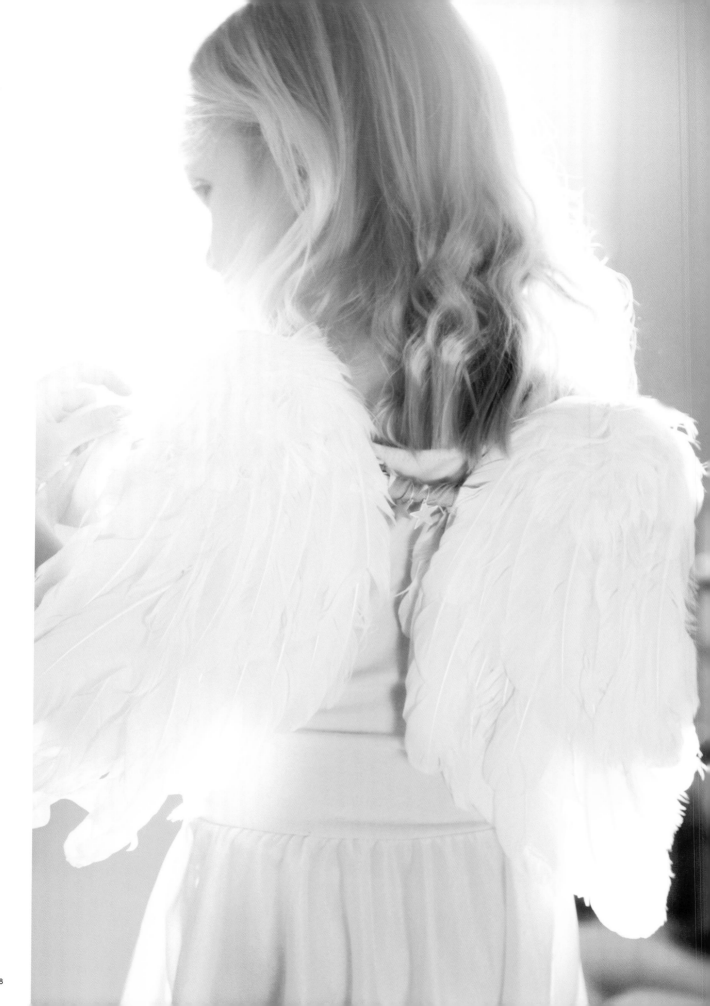

"I love to shop the boys' section at J. Crew for Chiara!"

—*Ramya Giangola,* **BRANDING CONSULTANT**

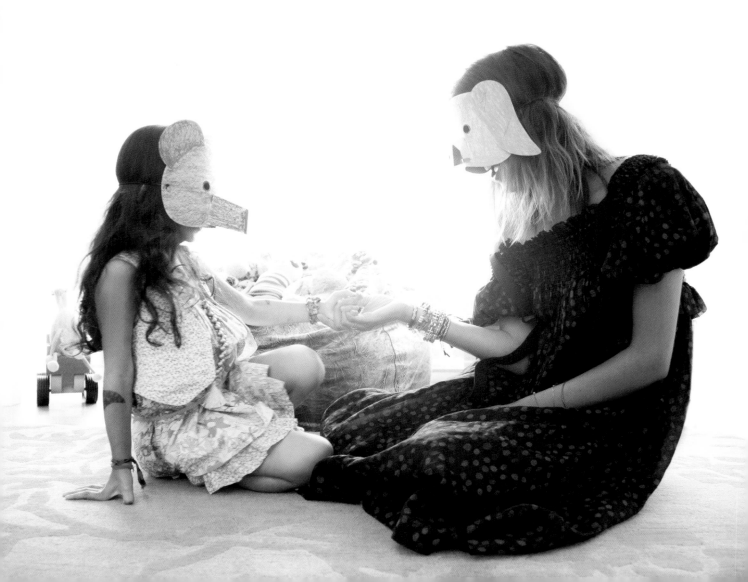

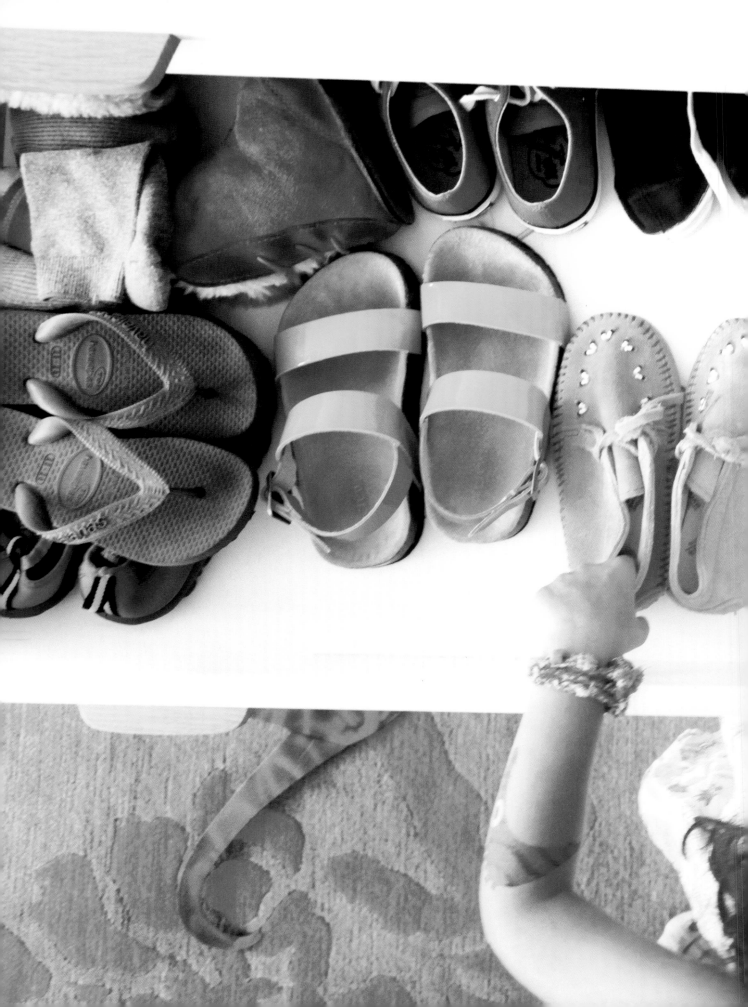

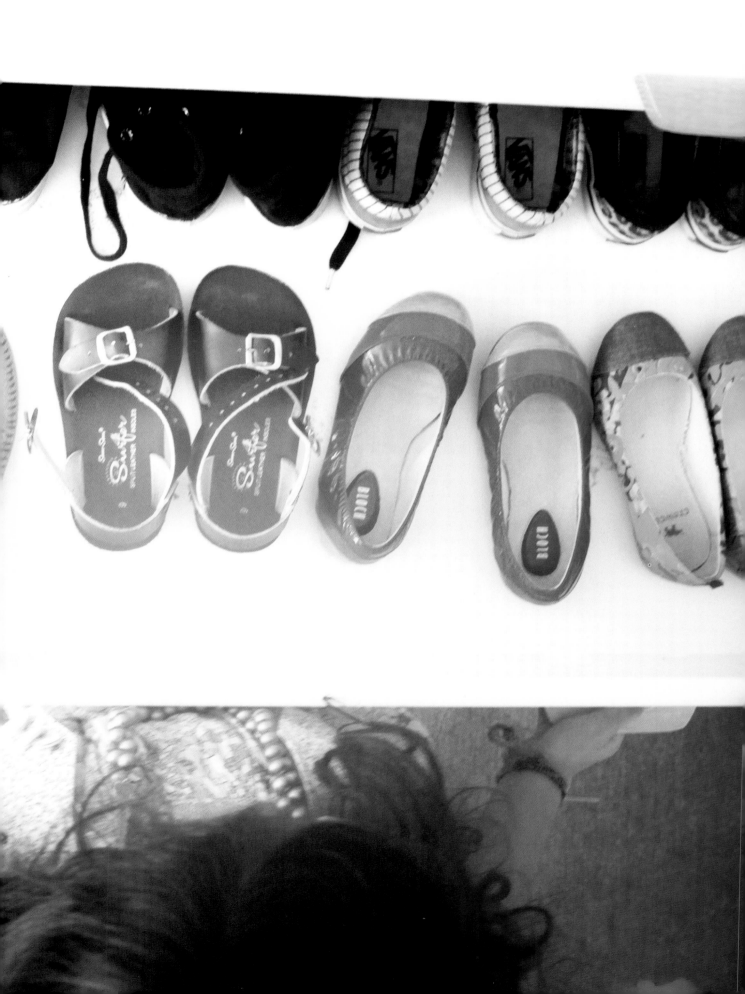

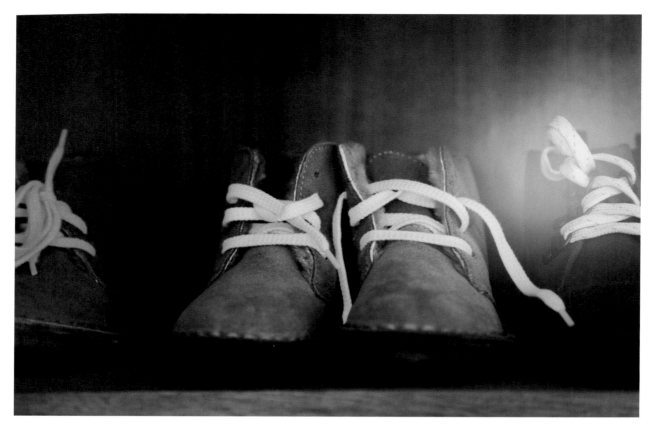

ABOVE: To add an unexpected pop of color to her son's neutral boots, Jenni Kayne replaced the standard laces with a variety of neon styles. BELOW: Instead of hiding these adorable beaded moccasins in her son's closet, Rachelle Hruska cleverly displays them on a shelf, instantly making them part of the room's eclectic décor.

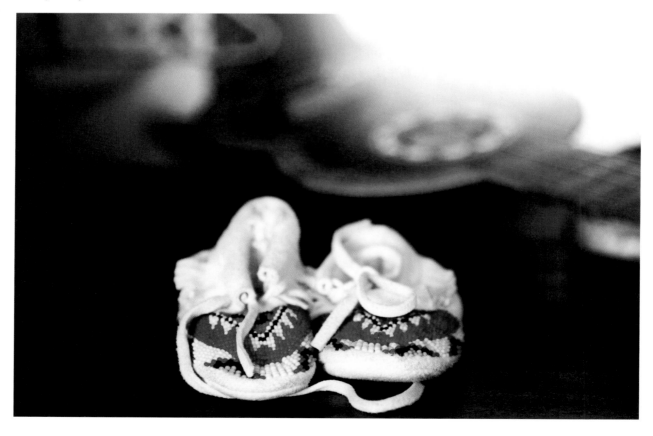

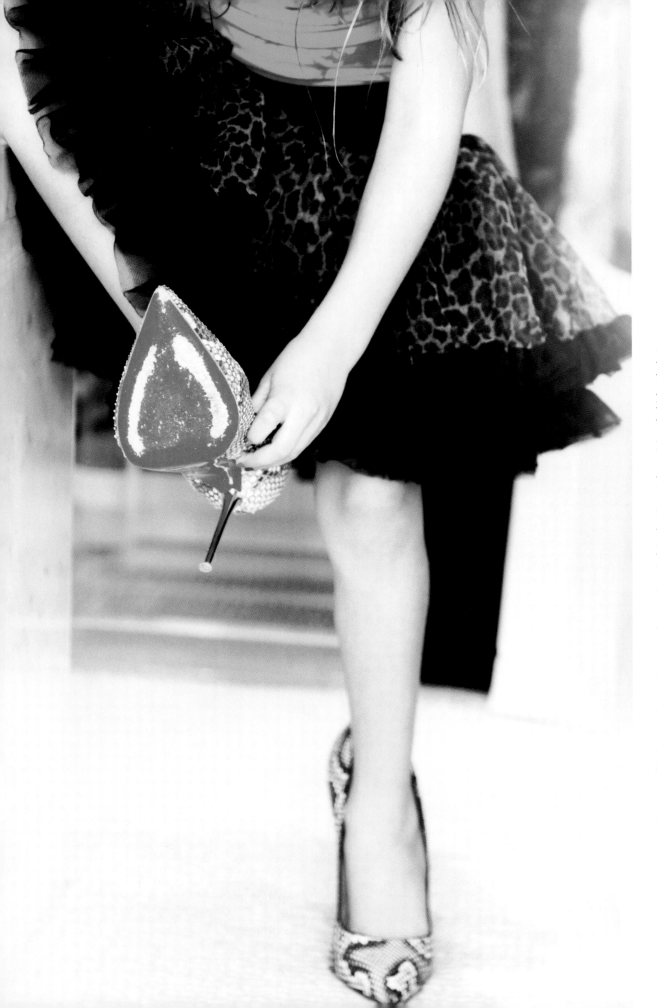

LEFT: Drew, Jennifer Fisher's super-stylish daughter, loves to dress up in her mom's six-inch Louboutins—in her opinion, the higher the better.

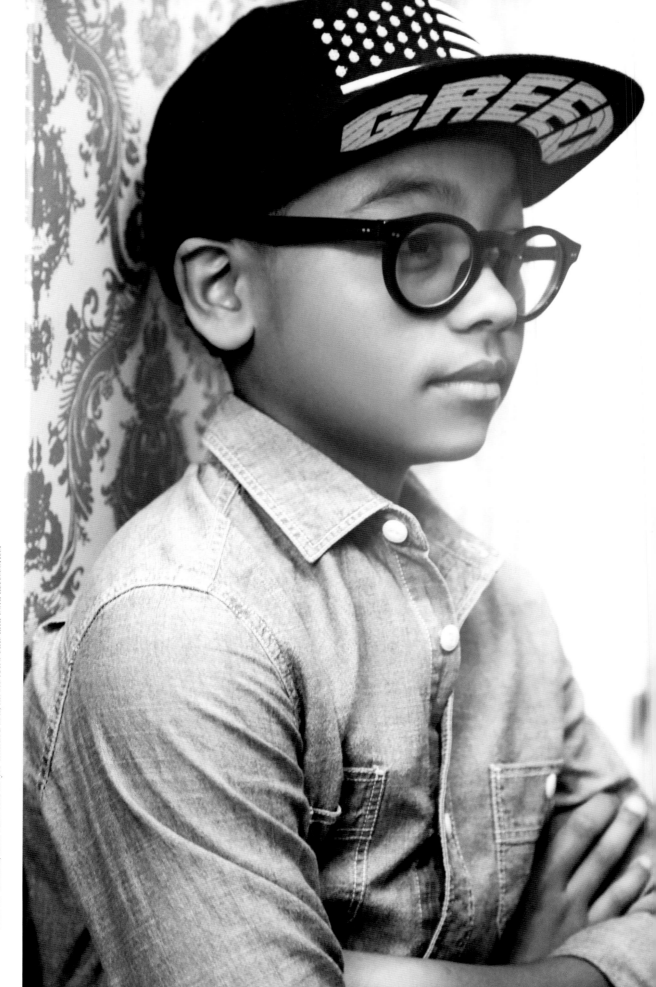

RIGHT: Chance, June Ambrose's style-minded son, favors retro cuts and bold accessories.

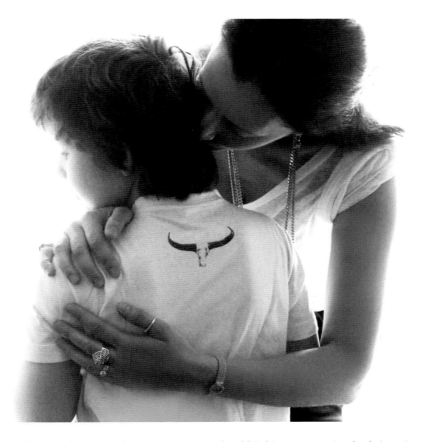

ABOVE: For her son Martin, Caroline Deroche Pasquier favors vintage pieces and artful T-shirts. BELOW: Jewelry designer Lynn Ban loves to dress her son Sebastian in black clothes and admits that "at birthday parties, people tell me they can always spot him because he's the only kid all in black."

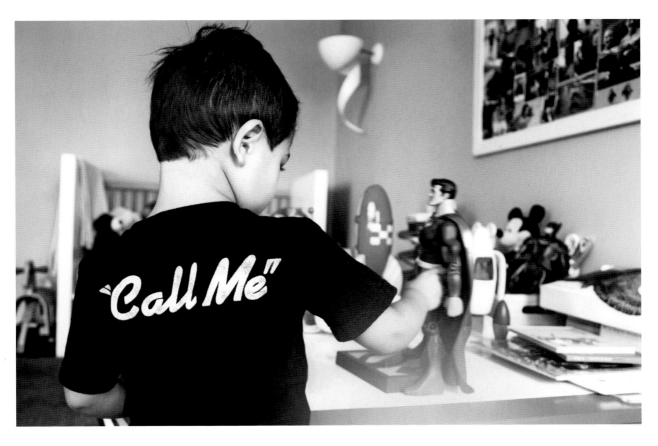

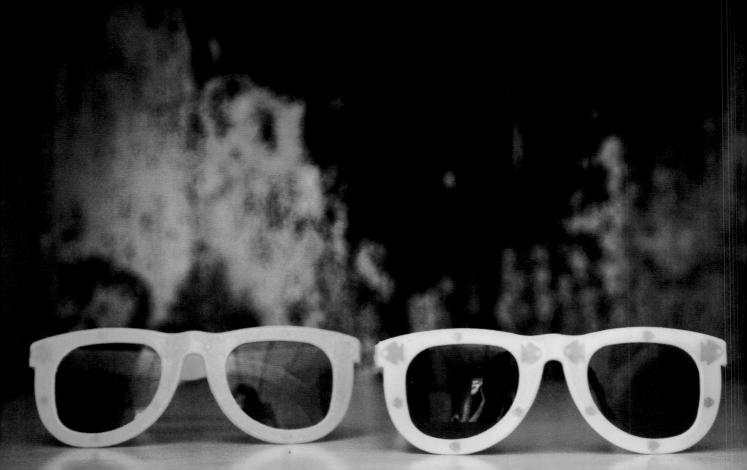

"She's starting to pick
out what she wears.
She'll say 'Elmo shirt!' and
I think to myself, 'Nooooo!'
Then again, it's fun to
see her dress herself . . .
I get to see little bits and
pieces of her creativity."

—Jeanann Williams, STYLIST

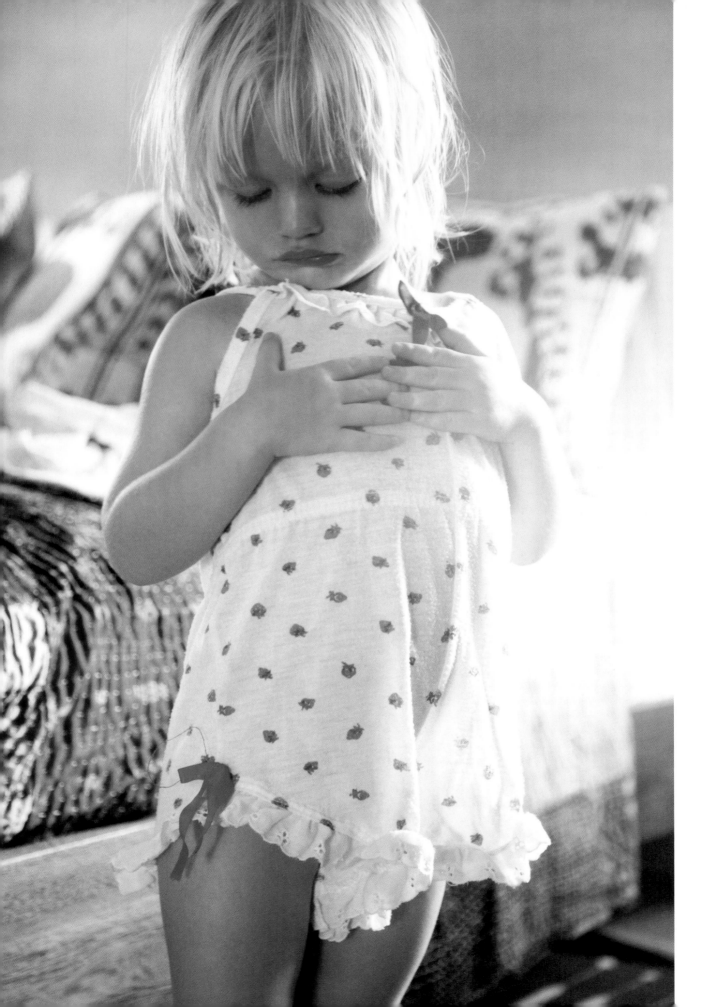

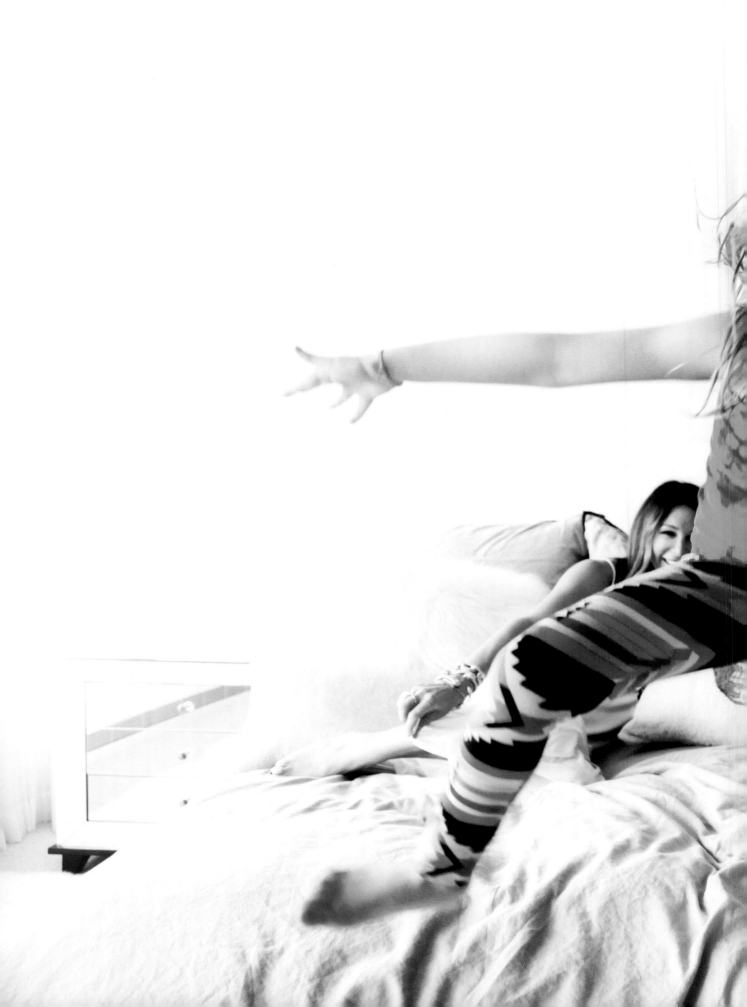

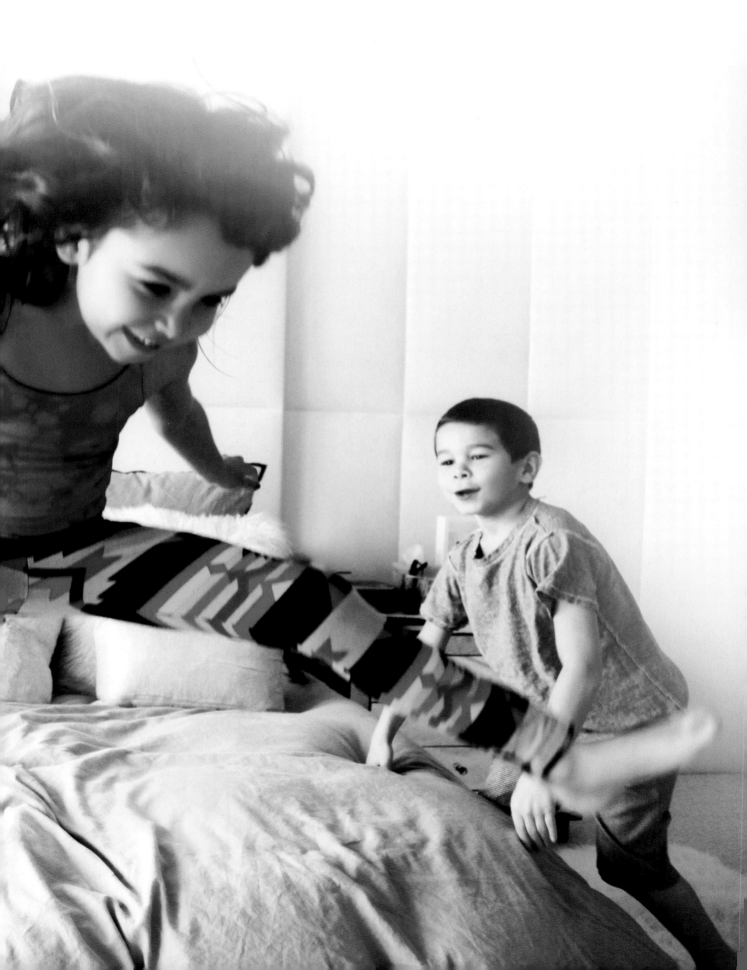

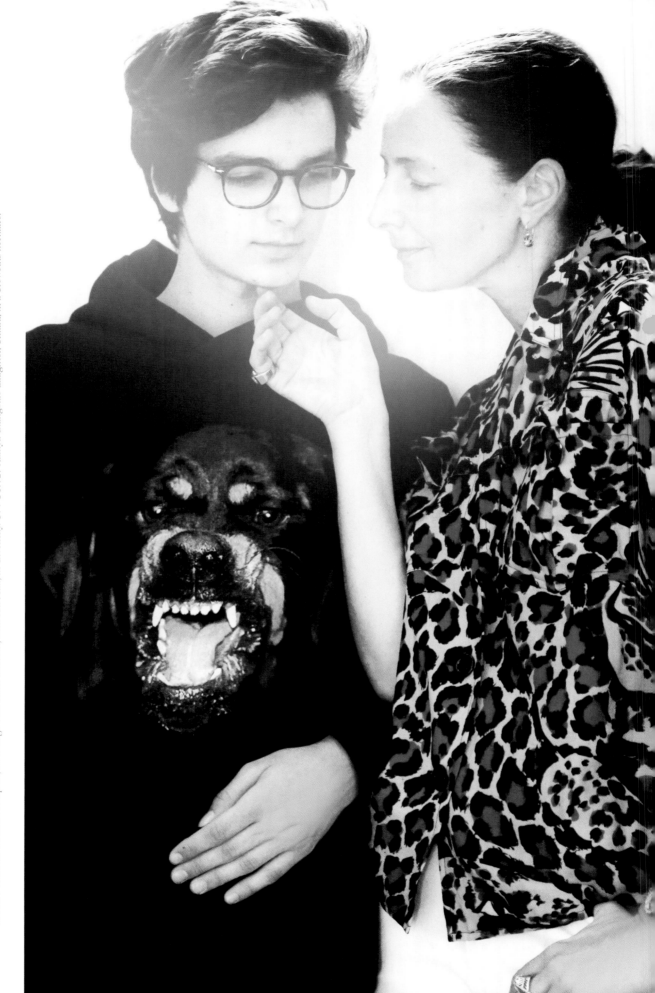

RIGHT: Caroline Deroche Pasquier, in vintage Yves Saint Laurent, with son Jean, in Givenchy. OPPOSITE: Ramya Giangola's daughter, Chiara, in a Crewcuts necklace.

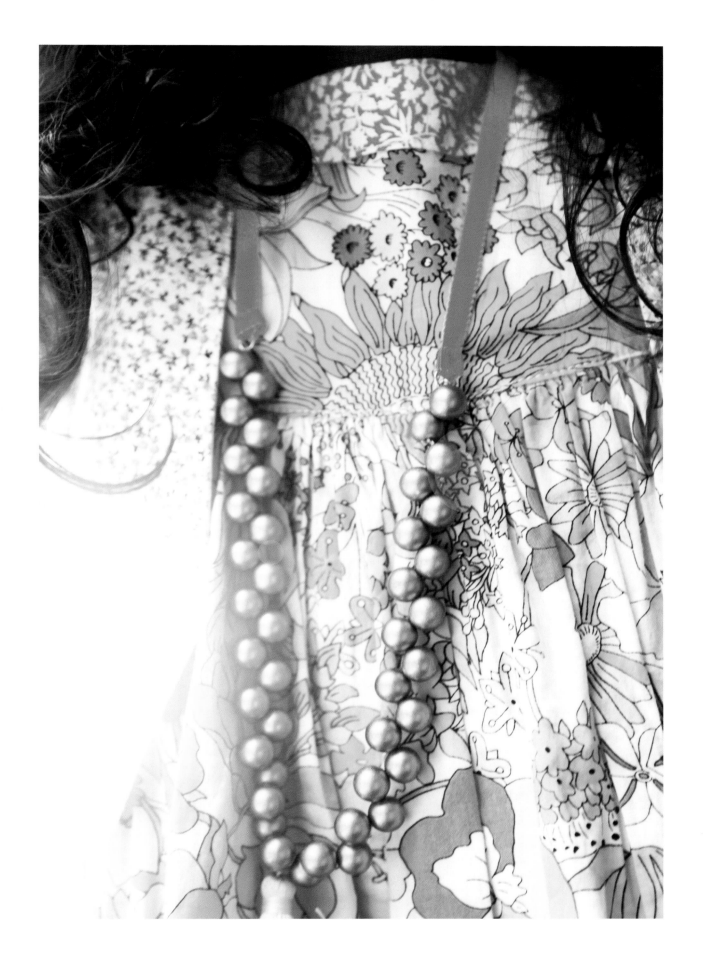

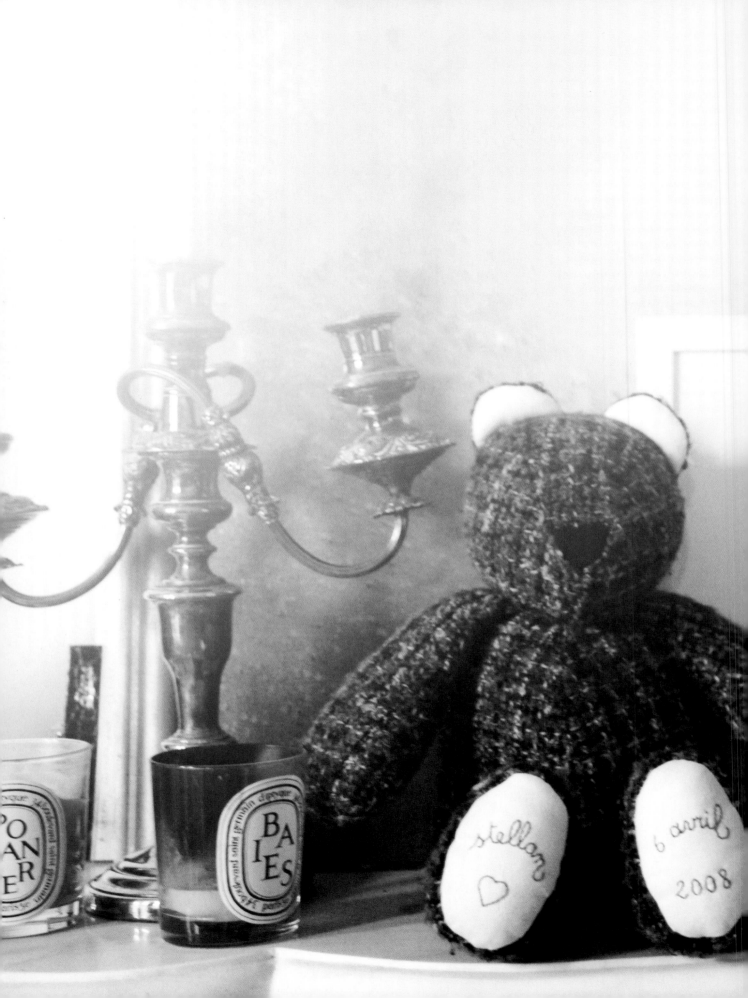

CHAPTER NINE

Inspiring Ideas

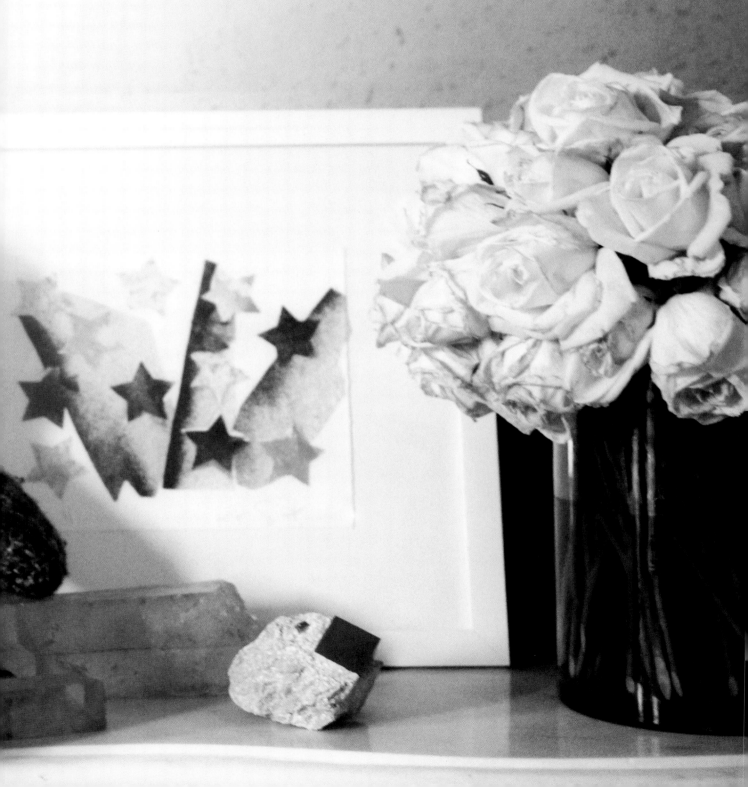

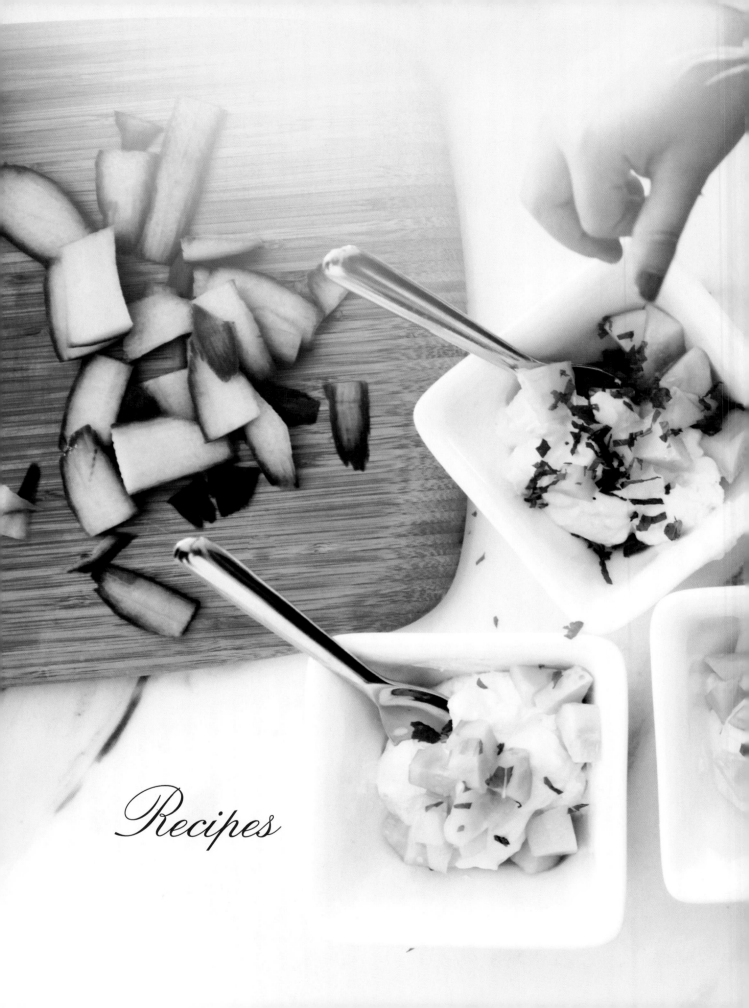

Recipes

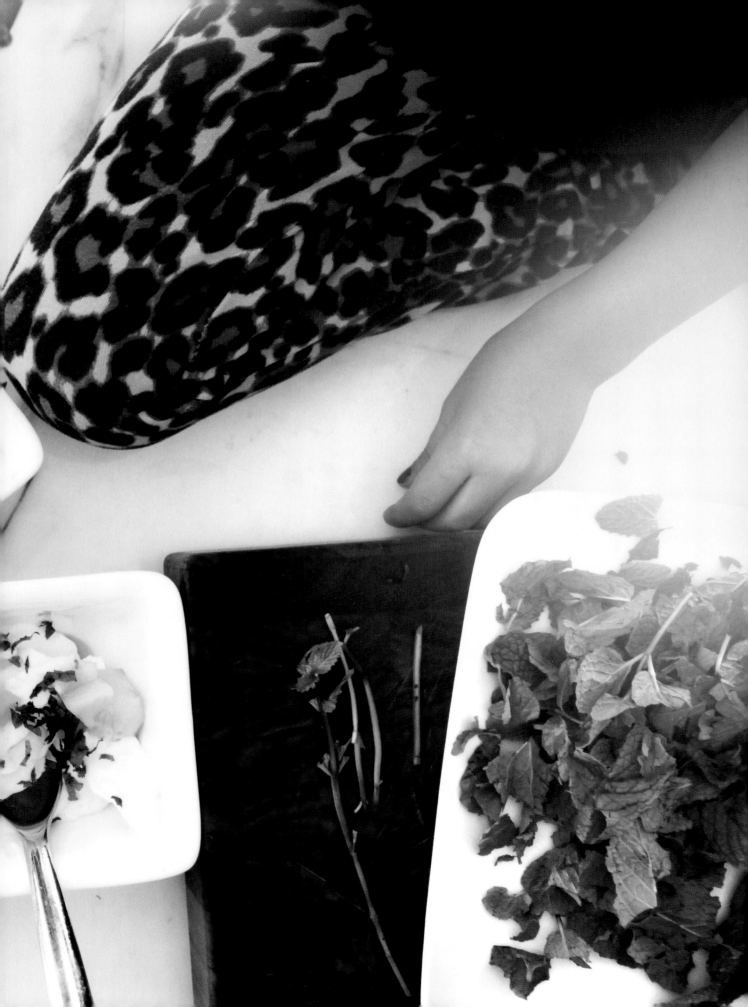

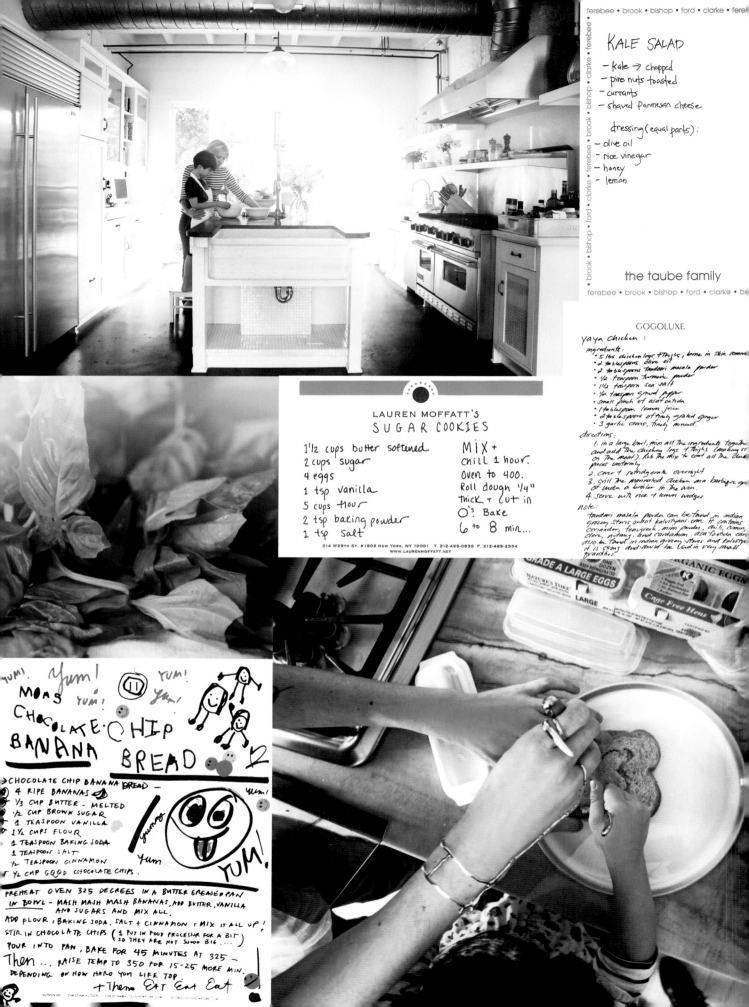

KALE SALAD

- kale → chopped
- pine nuts toasted
- currants
- shaved Parmesan cheese

dressing (equal parts):

- olive oil
- rice vinegar
- honey
- lemon

the taube family

GOGOLUXE

yaya chicken

ingredients:
- 5 lbs chicken legs + thighs, bone in skin remove
- 2 tablespoons olive oil
- 2 tablespoons tandoori masala powder
- 1/2 teaspoon turmeric powder
- 1 1/2 teaspoon sea salt
- 1/2 teaspoon ground pepper
- small pinch of asafoetida
- 1 tablespoon lemon juice
- 2 tablespoons of finely grated ginger
- 3 garlic cloves, finely minced.

directions:
1. In a large bowl, mix all the ingredients together and add the chicken legs + thighs (making sl on the meat). Rub the mix to coat all the chick pieces uniformly.
2. Cover + refrigerate overnight
3. Grill the marinated chicken on a barbeque gr or under a broiler in the oven.
4. Serve with rice + lemon wedges

note:
tandoori masala powder can be found in Indian grocery stores and at kalustyans.com. It contains coriander, fenugreek, mango powder, chili, cumin, clove, nutmeg, and cardamom. asafoetida can also be found in Indian grocery stores and kalustya It is strong and should be used in very small quantities.

LAUREN MOFFATT's
SUGAR COOKIES

1 1/2 cups butter softened	MIX +
2 cups sugar	chill 1 hour.
4 eggs	Oven to 400.
1 tsp vanilla	Roll dough 1/4"
5 cups flour	thick + cut in
2 tsp baking powder	O's Bake
1 tsp salt	6 to 8 min...

214 W 29TH ST. #1503 NEW YORK, NY 10001 T. 212-465-0839 F. 212-465-2334
WWW.LAURENMOFFATT.NET

YUM! Yum! YUM! MOAS Yum! Yum!

MOAS CHOCOLATE CHIP BANANA BREAD

→CHOCOLATE CHIP BANANA BREAD –
- 4 RIPE BANANAS
- 1/3 CUP BUTTER - MELTED
- 1/2 CUP BROWN SUGAR
- 1 TEASPOON VANILLA
- 1 1/2 CUPS FLOUR
- 1 TEASPOON BAKING SODA
- 1 TEASPOON SALT
- 1/2 TEASPOON CINNAMON
- 1/2 CUP GOOD CHOCOLATE CHIPS.

PREHEAT OVEN 325 DEGREES IN A BUTTER GREASED PAN
IN BOWL – MASH MASH MASH BANANAS, ADD BUTTER, VANILLA
AND SUGARS AND MIX ALL.
ADD FLOUR, BAKING SODA, SALT + CINNAMON + MIX IT ALL UP!
STIR IN CHOCOLATE CHIPS (I PUT IN FOOD PROCESSOR FOR A BIT)
SO THEY ARE NOT SWOO BIG....)
POUR INTO PAN, BAKE FOR 45 MINUTES AT 325 –
Then ... RAISE TEMP TO 350 FOR 15-25 MORE MIN.
DEPENDING ON HOW HARD YOU LIKE TOP.
+ Then EAT EAT EAT

YUM! Yum! Yum!

ELIZABETH STEWART

Whole Wheat Oatmeal Banana Pancakes

3/4 cup quick-cooking oats
1 1/2 cups buttermilk
3/4 cup whole wheat flour
1 1/2 tsp. baking powder
3/4 tsp. baking soda
1/2 tsp. cinnamon
1/8 tsp. grated nutmeg
1/2 tsp. salt
1 large egg
2 tablespoons melted butter
2 tablespoons packed brown sugar
1 banana, cut in small pieces

Soak oats in half the buttermilk. Meanwhile, lightly beat the egg and add the rest of the buttermilk, melted butter, oats mixture, sugar, then the rest of the dry ingredients. Mix just to combine. Heat a griddle to medium heat and work in batches. Use 1/4 cup batter per pancakes and press in banana pieces before flipping each pancake. Serve with warmed maple syrup.

F/E/Y/T

Baked Kale Chips

Ingredients:
bunch of kale
1 TBL of olive oil
1 tsp sea salt

Heat oven to 350. Line a non-insulated cookie sheet with parchment paper
Tear kale leaves into bite sized pieces (remove stems)
Wash and dry with a salad spinner
Drizzle kale with olive oil and sprinkle with salt to season

Bake until edges brown but are not burnt, 10 to 15 minutes.

FEYT 198 LAFAYETTE STREET 4TH FLOOR NEW YORK, NEW YORK 10012 212 941 5804 WWW.FEYT.COM

KATE YOUNG

Quiche

Crust
1 · 3/4 cup flour
1 stick butter
2 TB creme fraiche
1 egg
Mix flour + butter w/ some salt until it's all broken pieces the size of peas... Add creme fraiche + egg. Make 2 balls. Refrigerate 1 hour.

Filling
Sauté an onion + some kale, chard or spinach. Stir into 5 eggs, 3 TB creme fraiche, salt, pepper. A little nutmeg. Add grated cheddar. Pour into rolled out crust + bake for 45 mins at 375° x

---

Dwell Studio

PASTA + PEAS TWO WAYS FOR KIDDIE + FOODIES...

KIDS -
1 BOX PASTA (FUN SHAPE)
1/2 POUND PEAS SHELLED
3 TBS BUTTER
GRATED PARMESAN
(TOSS ALL TOGETHER WHEN COOKED)

FOR PARENTS —
ADD 3 HANDFULS OF CHOPPED ARUGULA
ZEST OF 1/2 LEMON
3 PIECES OF PROSCIUTTO (SAUTÉED LIKE BACON)
SALT + PEPPER TO TASTE

ENJOY! CHRISTIANE

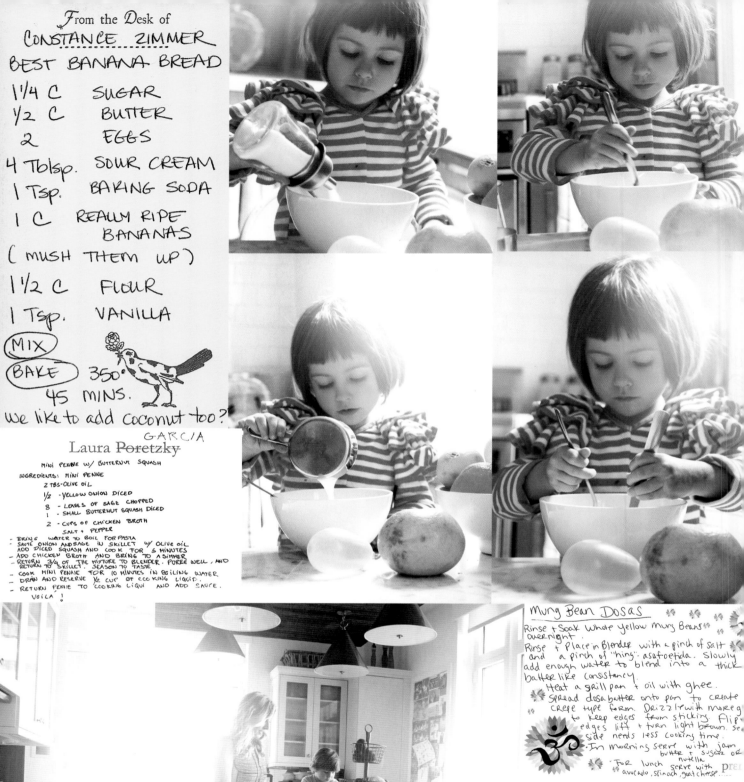

From the Desk of
CONSTANCE ZIMMER

BEST BANANA BREAD

1¼ C	SUGAR
½ C	BUTTER
2	EGGS
4 Tblsp.	SOUR CREAM
1 Tsp.	BAKING SODA
1 C	REALLY RIPE BANANAS (MUSH THEM UP)
1½ C	FLOUR
1 Tsp.	VANILLA

(MIX)
(BAKE) 350°
45 MINS.

we like to add coconut too?

Laura Poretzky GARCIA

Mini Penne w/ Butternut Squash

INGREDIENTS: MINI PENNE
2 TBS - OLIVE OIL
½ - YELLOW ONION DICED
8 - LEAVES OF SAGE CHOPPED
1 - SMALL BUTTERNUT SQUASH DICED
2 - CUPS OF CHICKEN BROTH
SALT + PEPPER

- BRING WATER TO BOIL FOR PASTA
- SAUTE ONION AND SAGE IN SKILLET W/ OLIVE OIL
- ADD DICED SQUASH AND COOK FOR 5 MINUTES
- ADD CHICKEN BROTH AND BRING TO A SIMMER
- RETURN ¾ OF THE MIXTURE TO BLENDER. PUREE WELL, AND RETURN TO SKILLET. SEASON TO TASTE
- COOK MINI PENNE FOR 10 MINUTES IN BOILING WATER.
- DRAIN AND RESERVE ½ CUP OF COOKING LIQUID.
- RETURN PENNE TO COOKING LIQUI AND ADD SAUCE.
VOILA !

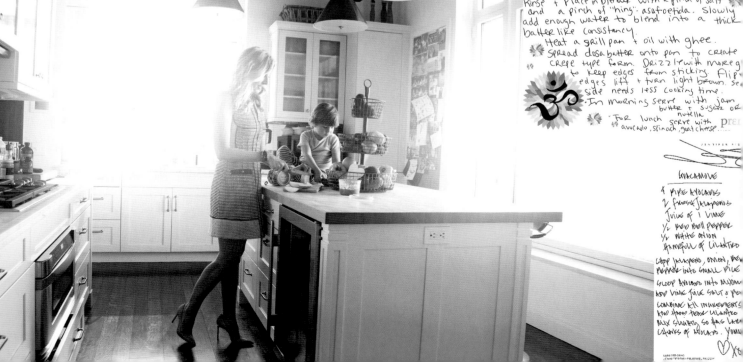

Mung Bean Dosas

Rinse + Soak Whole Yellow Mung Beans overnight.
Rinse + Place in Blender with a pinch of salt and a pinch of "hing" asafoetida. Slowly add enough water to blend into a thick batter like consistency.
Heat a grill pan + oil with ghee.
Spread dosa batter onto pan to create crepe type form. Drizzle with more ghee to keep edges from sticking. Flip edges lift + turn light brown. Second side needs less cooking time.
In morning serve with jam, butter + sugar or nutella.
For lunch serve with avocado, spinach, goat cheese...

GUACAMOLE

4 RIPE AVOCADOS
2 FRESH JALAPENOS
JUICE OF 1 LIME
½ RED BELL PEPPER
½ WHITE ONION
HANDFULL OF CILANTRO

CHOP JALAPENO, ONION, BELL PEPPER INTO SMALL DICE
SCOOP AVOCADO INTO MIXING
ADD LIME JUICE, SALT + PEPPER
COMBINE ALL INGREDIENTS
KEEP SOME FRESH CILANTRO
MIX SLIGHTLY SO HAS LARGE CHUNKS OF AVOCADO. YUMM!

MEXICAN CABBAGE SALAD

RED CABBAGE - 1
RED PEPPER - 1
RED OR WHITE ONION - 1
CILANTRO
MAYO
LEMON + LIME

CUT HALF A HEAD OF RED CABBAGE INT
_ IN. STRIPS. CUT PEPPER + ONION INTO HALF
_CH CUBES. CHOP CILANTRO. MIX EVERYTHING
_TO A BOWL. SEASON WITH ONE TABLE SPOON
_ MAYO, SALT, PEPPER AND LIME.

_ST EATEN WITH GUACAMOLE AND CHIPS !!!

Roast Potatoes

1) Small red potatoes
2) chop in half
3) place on tray w/ olive oil, salt and pepper, sprigs of rosemary
4) place in oven at like 350° til brown
5) 20 mins (?)
6) remove, push around and unstick.
7) put back in oven for like 10 mins

BY AIR MAIL
PAR AVION

10/10

SHEPARD'S PIE

4 lb LEAN GROUND BEEF
2 LARGE YELLOW ONIONS
4 CLOVES OF GARLIC
8 LARGE POTATOES PEELED + CUBED
1 CUP OF MILK
4 TABLESPOONS OF BUTTER
2 CANS DICED TOMATOES WITH HERBS
SALT & PEPPER TO TASTE

CHOP ONION INTO SMALL CUBES.
MINCE GARLIC. SAUTEE TOGETHER
UNTIL SOFT. MIX IN RAW BEEF
UNTIL LIGHT BROWN. MIX IN
DICED TOMATOES. COOK ON LOW
HEAT FOR 30-45 MIN.
ADD SALT & PEPPER.
BOIL CUT POTATOES UNTIL SOFT.
DRAIN + PUT BACK INTO POT. ADD
MILK + BUTTER. ADD SALT.
PUT MEAT MIXTURE IN CASSEROLE
DISH WITH POTATOES ON TOP.
BAKE 30-40MIN   AT 325°

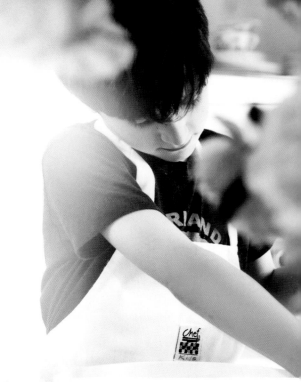

tibi

Lemon Ricotta Cookies with Lemon Glaze

· 2½ cup flour
· 1 teaspoon baking powder
· 2 eggs
· 1 (15 oz) Container whole milk ricotta cheese
· 1½ cups powdered sugar
· 1 teaspoon salt
· 1 stick unsalted butter
· 2 cups sugar
· 1 lemon, zested
· 3 tablespoons lemon juice

Directions:

Preheat oven to 375 degrees Farenheit
Cookies—
In medium bowl combine flour, baking powder and salt. Set aside.
In large bowl combine butter & sugar. Beat with an electric mixer until light & fluffy (3 min). Add eggs, one at time, beating until incorporated. Add ricotta cheese, lemon juice & lemon zest. Beat to combine. Stir in the dry ingredients.
Line 2 baking sheets with parchment paper. Spoon the dough (approx 2 tblspoons) onto sheets. Bake for 15 min. until golden at edges. Remove from oven & let cool for 20 min.
Glaze — Combine powder sugar, lemon juice & lemon zest in small bowl and stir until smooth. Spoon onto cookies.

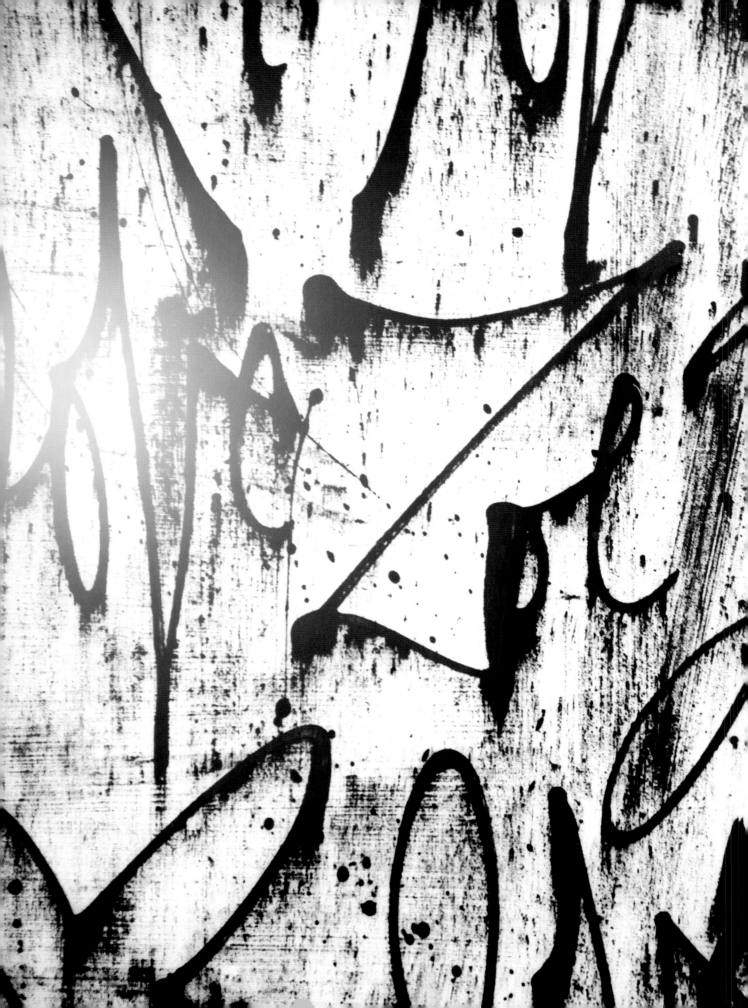

Names

Summer	Poppy	Chance	Bailey
Penelope	Rumi Joon	Sam	Luca Shai
Ava Harlow	Indi Joon	Sebastian	Eddie
Margot Rae	Tuesday	Leo	Jackson
Violet Marlowe	Frankie	Lazer	August
Secret	Kit Clementine	Arthur Saint	Harry
Mae	Gigi Clementine	Oliver	Liam
Cleo	Zoe	John	Casper
Bianca	Isabel	Gustav	Knox
Charlie	Ruby	Baron	Charlie
Zoe Lee	Zoey	Snowden	Oscar
Drew	Sydney	Jivan	Alastair
Georgiana	Anaïs	Jean	Stellan
Violet	Ella	Martin	Leif
Lowe	Sunny	Shane	Ben
Grayson	Ivy	Dashiel	Jonah
Ripley	Coco	Maxwell	Cassius
Mae	Birdie	Valentine	Gabriel
Rafaella	Chiara	Tanner	Bishop
Isabelle	Stella	Arthur	Ford
Luna	Ava Lily	William	Clarke
Esme	Delilah		
Wallis			

Resources

Acknowledgments

The making of this book has given us the ultimate lesson in creating balance. Over the course of our year-long journey planning, photographing, writing, designing, and editing this book, while working at our full-time jobs as photo director for Hearst Digital Media and InStyle.com senior fashion editor, we were also lucky enough to experience some of the most special moments of our lives—between the two of us, we renovated an apartment, got pregnant, planned a wedding, had a baby, got married, and went on a cross-country New Zealand honeymoon (not necessarily in that order). The angels we are lucky enough to call our family and friends carried us through to the finish line. They were the calm voice on the other end of the phone after countless long nights, early mornings, and busy weekends. We are blessed beyond belief.

Wendy, Ruby, Ray, Betty, Kathleen, Kim, Bridget, Melanie, Mary, and Eleanor—our beautiful mamas, sisters, grandmothers, and aunts: Quite simply, you are the reason this book exists. Your strength of spirit and ability to make motherhood look effortless inspired us to explore the idea of balance and the mind-blowing bond between mother and child. You are our rocks, our hearts, our souls.

There's not enough room on this page, or in this entire book for that matter, to give proper thanks to the saintly men in our lives, our husbands David and Anthony. You lived and breathed these 224 pages and experienced every high and low right along with us.

Your selflessness allowed us to put 1,000 percent into making this dream of ours come true. Your brilliance and wit are just the icing on the cake. You are the backbone of this book, and the loves of our lives.

To our wonderful editor, Rebecca, and the entire Abrams team: Thank you for believing in The Glow from day one, and convincing us that we were ready to take the leap from website to coffee table book. To our amazing literary agent, Kari, you held our hands and guided us with warmth and patience.

To the smart, powerful, hard-working women featured in this book, we give you our endless gratitude. You are our friends, our mentors, and a constant source of inspiration for us. Your insouciant style and eloquent honesty about modern motherhood have brought The Glow to life.

And to you, our dear readers, thank you for inspiring us every day. From the moment we hit "publish" on our very first post, you have embraced The Glow and believed in our content with your whole hearts. Your support, feedback, and wisdom have guided us every step of the way, and we thank you from the bottom of our hearts for letting us create this book for you.

A special thank-you to the newest and littlest member of The Glow team—baby Plum Lillian, thank you for teaching me what it feels like to wear my heart on the outside.

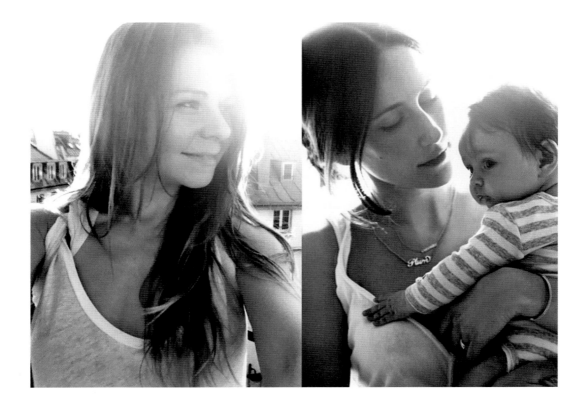

PAINTING BY *Jemima Kirke*

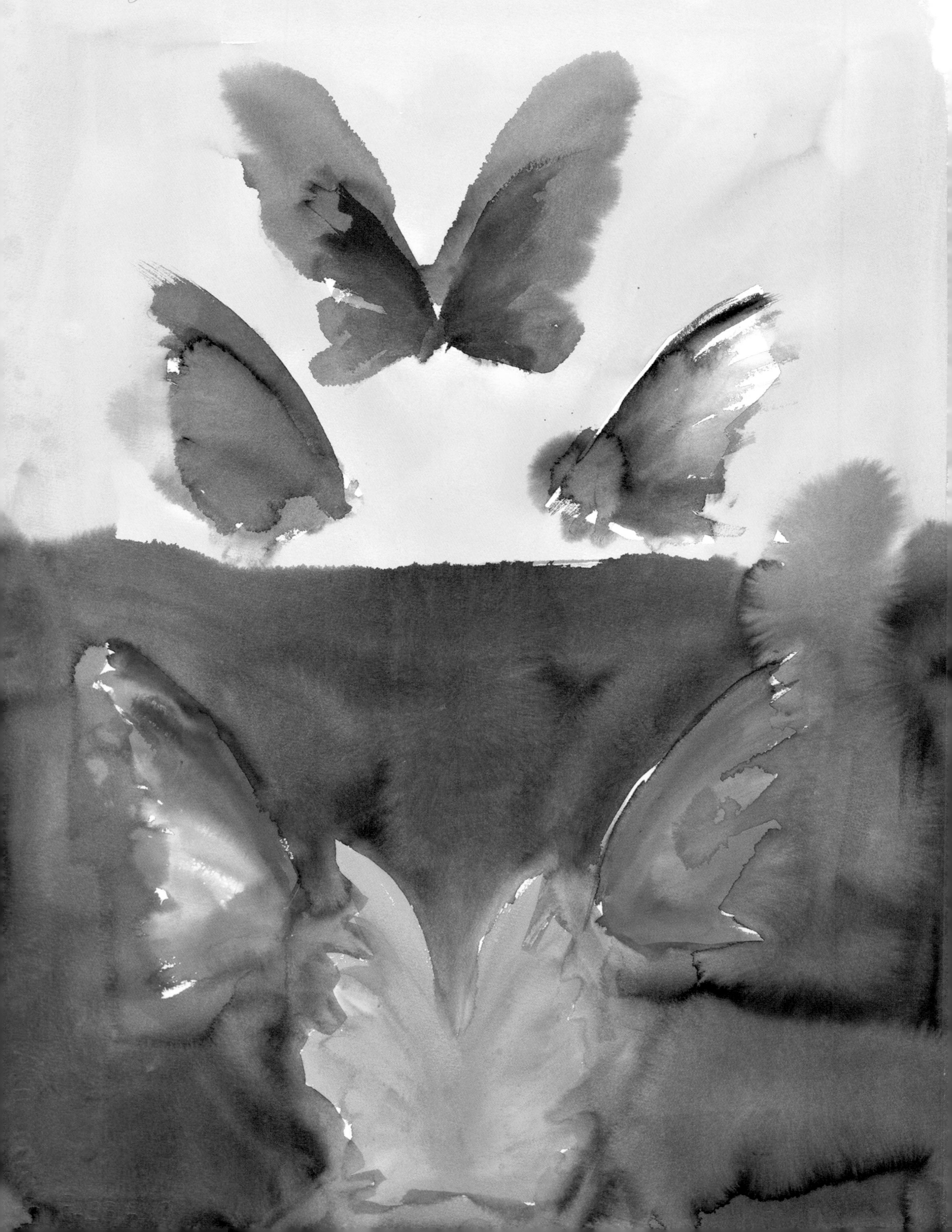